PTERYGIUM

TECHNIQUES AND TECHNOLOGIES FOR SURGICAL SUCCESS

PTERYGIUM

TECHNIQUES AND TECHNOLOGIES FOR SURGICAL SUCCESS

Edited by:

John A. Hovanesian, MD
Harvard Eye Associates
Laguna Beach, California
Clinical faculty
Jules Stein Eye Institute
University of California
Los Angeles, California

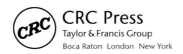

CRC Press
Taylor & Francis Group
Boca Raton London New York

CRC Press is an imprint of the
Taylor & Francis Group, an **informa** business

First published 2012 by SLACK Incorporated

Published 2024 by CRC Press
2385 NW Executive Center Drive, Suite 320, Boca Raton FL 33431

and by CRC Press
4 Park Square, Milton Park, Abingdon, Oxon, OX14 4RN

CRC Press is an imprint of Taylor & Francis Group, LLC

© 2012 Taylor & Francis Group, LLC

Library of Congress Cataloging-in-Publication Data

Pterygium : technqiues and technologies for surgical success / [edited by] John A. Hovanesian.
     p. ; cm.
  Includes bibliographical references and index.
  ISBN 978-1-55642-978-1 (pbk.)
 1. Pterygium--Surgery. I. Hovanesian, John A., 1967-
 [DNLM: 1. Pterygium--surgery. 2. Ophthalmologic Surgical Procedures--methods. WW 212]
 RE326.P7P74 2011
 617.7'1--dc23
                         2011012980

ISBN: 9781556429781 (pbk)
ISBN: 9781003526094 (ebk)

DOI: 10.1201/9781003526094

Dedication

For Mom, Dad, and Charles.

Contents

Acknowledgments

This book is the product of its individual chapter authors who agreed to contribute their knowledge and effort—despite many demands for their time—to better educate the ophthalmic community. We are all also indebted to their collaborators, fellows, and other trainees, both named and unnamed, who participated in research and writing.

It's been an inspiration to know Claes Dohlman, who kindly wrote this book's foreword and who has taught me and countless others a better understanding of the ocular surface through direct teaching, courses, and lectures.

Ken Kenyon and Michael Wagoner have each been personal influences on me, and with their first work on conjunctival autografts, have redefined pterygium surgery.

I first learned of sutureless methods for ocular surface surgery through Gabor Koranyi's publications, and I believe he deserves much credit for advancing the standard of care in these procedures.

David Hardten, Steven Kaufman, and Amar Agarwal deserve special mention because of their unending contributions to our courses and teaching efforts since 2005. Scheffer Tseng, although unable to contribute to this book, has also contributed greatly to the understanding of the eye's surface and has been a valued collaborator on our many courses at the American Academy of Ophthalmology (AAO) and the American Society of Cataract and Refractive Surgery (ASCRS).

My partners and associates in practice—Roger Ohanesian, Ed Kim, Diana Kersten, Paul Park, Jeff Jacobs, Nicki Stefanidis, and Karen Skvarna—have all been outstanding collaborators over the years, sharing their clinical experiences and support. Their continued friendship has been a delight.

In my fellowship at the UCLA Jules Stein Eye Institute, I was and still am appreciative of the teachings of Robert Maloney, Bart Mondino, Gary Holland, and Ella Factorovich, who helped me perform my first pterygium excisions with conjunctival autografts. Those who were my early teachers at Henry Ford Health Systems in Detroit all deserve much credit and include Con McCole (sadly now deceased), Dave Carey, Dan Steen, Howard Neff, Dave Bogorad, Julian Nussbaum, Bob Lesser, Murray Christianson, Uday Desai, Paul Edwards, Tom Byrd, Barry Skarf, Brian Bachynski, Pat Dennehy, and others.

My wife Tanya deserves special credit for her patience and understanding with the demands of publishing, even of this small text. I appreciate her saintly understanding of my absences so that this and other teaching works could go on.

Much gratitude also goes to Jennifer Briggs and John Bond from SLACK Incorporated, who have provided advice, support, and many hours of work. Peter Slack, Joan-Marie Stiglich, and Dave Mullin also have my gratitude for their collaboration since 2005 in publishing educational materials for eye care professionals. It's always been a pleasure to work with them.

Finally, it's appropriate to thank the patients of the book's contributors. Their continued trust and confidence, their referrals, and their willingness to participate in research studies have made all of our work possible.

About the Editor

John A. Hovanesian, MD is a member of the clinical faculty at the UCLA Jules Stein Eye Institute in Los Angeles, CA and is in private ophthalmic practice in Laguna Hills, CA with Harvard Eye Associates. He completed his undergraduate training in 3 years in the honors chemistry program at the University of Michigan in Ann Arbor, where he was a James B. Angell Scholar and was inducted into the Phi Beta Kappa honor society as a sophomore. After graduating Summa Cum Laude, he earned his medical degree from the University of Michigan Medical School and completed his residency training at Henry Ford Hospital in Detroit, MI, where he was named Resident of the Year and was selected by his faculty to serve as chief resident. He then completed a 2-year fellowship in cornea and external disease at the UCLA Jules Stein Eye Institute. In his private practice in Southern California, he directs one of the country's most recognized FDA study centers, evaluating new eye care technologies. He serves as a board member or consultant for over 20 eye technology companies.

As the son of two teachers, Dr. Hovanesian enjoys contributing to ophthalmic education and serves the American Academy of Ophthalmology as editor of the Online News and Education Network's cataract and anterior segment section. He is a regular contributor and member of the editorial board for *Ocular Surgery News*, *Cataract and Refractive Surgery Today*, *The Premier Surgeon*, *Advanced Ocular Care*, and *Primary Care Optometry News*. He blogs at http://www.osnsupersite.com/blog/hovanesian.aspx.

In his spare time, Dr. Hovanesian, an Eagle Scout, is a volunteer leader with the Boy Scouts of America serving as both cubmaster of his son's Cub Scout group and executive board member of the Orange County, California Council. He and his wife also teach Sunday school at his church in Costa Mesa, CA.

Contributing Authors

Amar Agarwal, MS, FRCS, FRCOphth (Chapter 10)
Director & Head of Department
Dr Agarwal's Eye Hospital & Eye Research Centre
Chennai, India

M. Camille Almond, MD (Chapter 5)
Cornea Fellow
University of Minnesota
Department of Ophthalmology
Minneapolis, Minnesota

Juan F. Batlle, MD (Chapter 6)
Professor and Chief
Ophthalmology Department
Hospital Dr. Elias Santana and Satellites Clinics
President, Centro Laser
President, Centro de Microgirugía Ocular y Láser
Multi-specialty Ophthalmology Ambulatory Surgery Center
Santo Domingo, Dominican Republic

Andrew S. Behesnilian, MD (Chapter 9)
Resident Physician in Urology
UCLA Medical Center
Los Angeles, California

Jay C. Bradley, MD (Chapter 11)
Assistant Professor
Cornea, External Disease, & Refractive Surgery, Cataract & Anterior Segment Surgery
Department of Ophthalmology & Visual Sciences
Texas Tech University Health Sciences Center
Lubbock, Texas

Hyung Cho, MD (Chapter 8)
Department of Ophthalmology
Albert Einstein College of Medicine
Montefiore Medical Center
Bronx, New York

Roy S. Chuck, MD, PhD (Chapter 8)
Department of Ophthalmology
Albert Einstein College of Medicine
Montefiore Medical Center
Bronx, New York

Jeanie Jin Yee Chui, MBBS, PhD (Chapter 1)
Postdoctoral Research Fellow
School of Medical Sciences
Department of Pathology
University of New South Wales
Kensington, New South Wales, Australia

Minas Theodore Coroneo, FRANZCO, MD, FRACS, MS (Chapter 1)
Professor of Ophthalmology
Prince of Wales Clinical School
Department of Ophthalmology
Prince of Wales Hospital
Randwick, New South Wales, Australia

B. Travis Dastrup, MD (Chapter 5)
Cornea Fellow
University of Minnesota
Department of Ophthalmology
Minneapolis, Minnesota

Mark A. Fava, MD, FRCSC (Chapter 3)
Boston Eye Group
Attending Surgeon, Beth Israel Deaconess Hospital
Boston, Massachusetts

Contributing Authors

Jane Fishler, MD (Chapter 7)
Ophthalmology Resident
Bascom Palmer Eye Institute
University of Miami
Miller School of Medicine
Miami, Florida

David R. Hardten, MD (Chapter 4)
Adjunct Associate Professor, Ophthalmology
University of Minnesota
Director of Research, Refractive Surgery & Fellowships
Minnesota Eye Consultants
Minneapolis, Minnesota

Richard H. Hoft, MD (Chapter 2)
Clinical Associate Professor, Ophthalmology
David Geffen School of Medicine at UCLA
Assistant Chief, Division of Ophthalmology
Los Angeles County/Harbor-UCLA Medical Center
Torrance, California

R. Duncan Johnson, MD (Chapter 2)
Clinical Instructor
Cornea and Uveitis Division, Department of Ophthalmology
David Geffen School of Medicine at UCLA
Los Angeles, California

Stephen C. Kaufman, MD, PhD (Chapter 5)
Lyon Professor of Ophthalmology
Director, Cornea and Refractive Surgery
University of Minnesota
Department of Ophthalmology
Minneapolis, Minnesota

Kenneth R. Kenyon, MD (Chapter 3)
Associate Clinical Professor, Ophthalmology
Harvard Medical School
Senior Clinical Scientist
Schepens Eye Research Institute
Cornea Consultants International
Boston, Massachusetts

Dhivya Ashok Kumar, MD (Chapter 10)
Consultant
Dr Agarwal's Eye Hospital & Eye Research Centre
Chennai, India

Vicky C. Pai, MD (Chapter 2)
Ophthalmic Surgeon
Jules Stein Eye Institute
University of California
Los Angeles, California

Victor L. Perez, MD (Chapter 7)
Associate Professor, Ophthalmology
Microbiology and Immunology
Bascom Palmer Eye Institute
University of Miami
Miller School of Medicine
Miami, Florida

Mohamed Abou Shousha, MD (Chapter 7)
Clinical Instructor, Cornea Service
Bascom Palmer Eye Institute
University of Miami
Miller School of Medicine
Miami, Florida

Preface

My partners in practice and I began exploring sutureless techniques with fibrin sealant in pterygium/conjunctival autograft surgery in 2003 after reading about Dr. Gabor Koranyi's success in Sweden. Like Dr. Koranyi, we found much less pain and shorter surgery than with sutures, and we began a formal study of our outcomes. Among sufferers of pterygium, word of that study—which I presented at the 2005 World Cornea Congress in Washington, DC—spread via Internet chat rooms and Web sites. Soon we all began seeing patients from far away places seeking more painless relief from their pterygia. Patients repeatedly told us that, upon their inquiry with nearby practices, no doctors in their local towns were familiar with tissue adhesive pterygium methods. By necessity, we learned how to "examine" patients postoperatively with emailed digital photographs. We monitored intraocular pressure remotely with the help of cooperative local practitioners. Those patients referred others, and soon we found ourselves with a pterygium referral practice.

I wanted to share these techniques with others and began organizing an ocular surface surgery course to be presented at the 2005 symposium of the American Society of Cataract and Refractive Surgery and the American Academy of Ophthalmology. Scheffer Tseng, Steve Kaufman, David Hardten, and Gabor Koranyi kindly agreed to join me as co-faculty in our first courses. High attendance prompted us to continue teaching the subject, and by 2008 we asked Amar Agarwal to join us in teaching his innovative "glued IOL" technique. Continuing to teach this course with these "giants" in ocular surgery has been one of the high points of my career.

Around 2007, I became intrigued with the powerful anti-inflammatory and antifibrotic properties of amniotic membrane for treating nonhealing corneal ulcers and managing bullous keratopathy. As a substitute for conjunctival autografts, amnion produced a slightly higher recurrence rate in my own hands. However, using the technique described in Chapter 9, I found amnion to be a powerful antifibrotic adjunct that augmented the recurrence-suppressing effects of conjunctival autografts, yielding a lower rate of recurrence. Increasingly, I have come to trust this technique for the eradication of more challenging pterygia.

All of the contributors to this book have been improving the standard of care for pterygium surgery and hope to see ongoing improvements in both the science described here and the ways we teach it. We all welcome the input and suggestions of readers for future editions and wish our colleagues success in putting this information into clinical practice.

John A. Hovanesian, MD
Harvard Eye Associates
Laguna Beach, California
Clinical Faculty
Jules Stein Eye Institute
University of California
Los Angeles, California

Foreword

The authors should be congratulated for a sharply focused, deep-probing text on a small but important slice of ophthalmology: the pterygium. This ocular surface phenomenon, which can range from a mild nuisance to a visual disaster, requires specialized expertise. This text should provide the ocular surface surgeon with all of the information necessary to deal with this tricky, elusive, often recurring problem. Dr. Hovanesian is a well-known expert on corneal and refractive problems and is highly qualified to be the leader and editor of this effort. The fame of his collaborators is a further guarantee for quality. This text will be the last word on the pterygium topic and, hopefully, will be updated in the future with further editions.

Claes H. Dohlman, MD
Former Chairman
Founder of Cornea Service
Emeritus Professor of Ophthalmology
Harvard Medical School
Boston, Massachusetts

Introduction

This text is written for eye surgeons who want to learn the latest techniques in order to improve their results with pterygium surgery, reduce the unpleasantness of postoperative pain, and eliminate the risk of recurrence. Until the mid to late 1990s, most residencies across the country taught bare sclera pterygium excision, sometimes using adjunctive radiation, Thio-TEPA, or the use of other antimetabolites. These early approaches—and a discussion of pterygium's pathogenesis—are discussed in Chapters 1 and 2. Antimetabolites continue to hold value as adjuncts in more modern graft surgery, but when combined with bare sclera surgery, they simply did not work well. The recurrences that invariably occurred were painful and harder to manage than the primary disease itself. Many who still use some variation of these techniques are reluctant to offer surgery to their pterygium patients, instead advising that continued lubrication is the safest course of action. This approach is no longer necessary.

Thanks to the early explorers of ocular surface reconstruction at the Massachusetts Eye and Ear Infirmary and elsewhere, we came to an understanding two decades ago that covering the defect created by pterygium excision could allow quiet healing. Further work with amniotic membrane as a tissue substitute and substrate for healing has expanded our surgical options; simplified our surgical approach; and provided an antifibrotic, anti-inflammatory adjunct with the safety of "mother's milk." Finally, the growing use of tissue sealants has expedited surgery and made healing virtually painless. These varied techniques and materials are discussed in Chapters 3 through 9, while Chapters 10 and 11 focus on the special topic of managing complications, most notably pterygium recurrence.

Some of these same techniques have been helpful in managing conjunctival chalasis, a disorder of conjunctival laxity that frequently causes ocular pain and is frequently mistaken for dry eye. Because this disorder is fairly common and shares many concepts with pterygium surgery, we include it with this text (Chapter 12).

Until we can better understand the pathogenesis of pterygium and reduce its incidence, we will continue to pursue better surgical techniques. Until then, it is the hope of its contributors that this book will help more surgeons adopt these tried-and-true techniques and make better surgical outcomes more widely available to our patients.

Pterygium Pathogenesis, Actinic Damage, and Recurrence

Jeanie Jin Yee Chui, MBBS, PhD and
Minas Theodore Coroneo, FRANZCO, MD, FRACS, MS

Pterygium, perhaps the most obvious of the ophthalmohelioses (sun-related eye diseases)[1,2] has proven to be an ophthalmic enigma.[3] It is potentially the Cinderella ocular disease—considered a diminutive condition and previously described as a degenerative condition. Increased understanding of its pathogenesis holds the key to further improvement in treatment modalities and outcomes. There is now strong evidence that ultraviolet (UV) light plays a major role in its development[4-6] and this is consistent with early evidence of an association with skin malignancy.[7] The likely involvement of both corneal epithelial stem cells and nerves provides an interesting model for their interaction with UV radiation in a transparent tissue. The active processes unleashed include inflammation, tissue invasion and degradation, angiogenesis, fibrosis, proliferation and apoptosis with involvement of matrix metalloproteinases (MMPs), cytokines, and growth factors (GFs). The presence of an inflammatory mass on the ocular surface may predispose the patient to a "pseudo-dry eye syndrome."[8] A better understanding of the molecular biology of this disease may result in the development of better medical treatments and may provide some insight as to why surgery sometimes fails.

The recognition that reflected, scattered light is critical in determining ocular exposure has helped to explain in part why high prevalence is not confined to the traditional peri-equatorial "pterygium-belt." The high reflectance of snow explains why pterygium is prevalent in arctic environments where incident light levels are relatively low. Pterygium prevalence varies considerably, and in addition to environmental factors there may also be individual susceptibility factors at play. In Australia, prevalence of up to 15% has been reported.[9] The Blue Mountains Eye Study, while finding a prevalence of up to 7%, reported pinguecula in up to 70% of the population.[10] The cost of managing pterygium both medically and surgically adds considerable cost to a nation's health budget.[11]

Hovanesian JA. *Pterygium: Techniques and Technologies for Surgical Success (pp 1-26).*

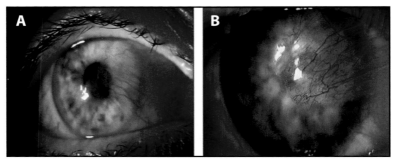

Figure 1-1. Clinical appearance of (A) primary and (B) recurrent pterygia.

Clinical Appearance and Histological Changes

Pterygium

Pterygia are wing-shaped ocular surface lesions extending from the bulbar conjunctiva onto the cornea (Figure 1-1). Pterygia occur predominantly on the nasal limbus, although temporal pterygia rarely occur in isolation.[12] Histologically, pterygia are characterized by centripetal growth of a leading edge of altered limbal epithelial cells followed by a squamous metaplastic epithelium with goblet cell hyperplasia and an underlying stroma of activated, proliferating fibroblasts; neovascularization; inflammatory cells; and extracellular matrix (ECM) remodeling (Figure 1-2). Based on the predominant histological features, pterygia have been divided into 3 types: proliferative, fibromatous, and atrophic sclerotic types.[13]

Pinguecula

The more common pinguecula appear as a yellow-white nodule on the nasal conjunctiva that does not cross the limbus. Whilst most pinguecula have a benign course, some may evolve into pterygia (Figure 1-3). Light and electron microscopic studies suggest that pingueculae share similar histological features to pterygia, including alterations in collagen and elastic fibers[14] and resembled fibrotic or early atrophic sclerotic pterygia.[13]

Pseudopterygium

Pseudopterygia are morphologically different compared to UV-induced pterygia in that they grow outside of the 3- and 9-o'clock positions and have a broad, flat leading edge.[15] Pseudopterygia may be triggered by ocular trauma,[16-18] previous surgery,[19,20] or chemical exposure.[21] It is suggested that pseudopterygia may be related to keloids, given that they share similar histological features of densely packed collagen and mixed chronic inflammatory infiltrate.[17]

Epidemiology

Pterygium is an ocular surface disease that affects human populations around the world. Depending on the age and racial groups examined, the prevalence of pterygium

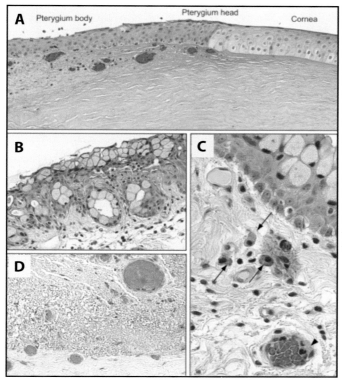

Figure 1-2. Hematoxylin- and Eosin-stained paraffin sections of pterygia. (A) A leading edge of corneal-like epithelium at the head of the pterygium abruptly transitions into conjunctival-like epithelium over the body of the pterygium. (B) Goblet cell hyperplasia in the epithelium overlying the body of a pterygium. The pterygium stroma consists of (A) invading fibroblasts and blood vessels, (C, arrows) mast cells and (C, arrowhead) neutrophils, and altered ECM including dissolution of (A) Bowman's membrane and (D) elastosis. Original magnification x200 for A, x400 for B and D, and x1000 oil for C.

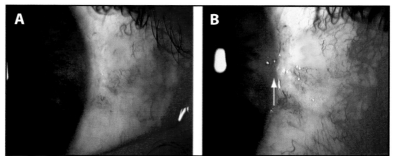

Figure 1-3. (A) Pinguecula transitioning into (B) a pterygium. Arrow indicates blood vessels crossing the limbus into the peripheral cornea.

varies from 0% to 56% (Table 1-1). The incidence of pterygium is positively associated with lifetime sun exposure[9,22,23] and other risk factors such as increasing age, male gender, and rural residency, whilst wearing glasses or a hat has been shown to have a protective effect.[24-27] More recently, chronic arsenic exposure has also been identified as an independent risk factor for pterygium.[28] One group reported a weak association with smoking,[29] but others found no association.[30] Elevated blood pressure and cholesterol levels were also observed to be associated with pterygium,[29] but the mechanism for this remains unclear. Pterygia are more common in some occupational groups such as welders, laborers, and those that work outdoors,[26,31,32] which reflects a key role of environmental exposure in the pathogenesis of this disease.

TABLE 1-1. GLOBAL PREVALENCE OF PTERYGIA BY GEOGRAPHIC LOCATION (POPULATION-BASED SURVEYS ONLY)

GEOGRAPHIC LOCATION	POPULATION GROUP	SAMPLE SIZE	AGE (YEARS)	% PREVALENCE OVERALL (RANGE)	STUDY
Mainland, Australia	Aboriginals Nonaboriginals	64314 40799	0-60+	3.41 (0.25-15.3) 1.11 (0.04-12)	Moran & Hollows[9]
Blue Mountains, New South Wales, Australia	Mixed	3564	49-80+	7.3	Panchapakesan et al[10]

Melbourne, Victoria, Australia	Mixed
	  Urban
	  Nursing homes
	  Rural
		
		3229
		403
		1473
			40-90+	
				1.2
				1.7
				6.7
					McCarty et al[33]

North Island, New Zealand	Maoris (rural)	333	0-80+	2.7	Mann & Potter[34]
Rarotonga, Cook Islands	Polynesians (rural)	986	20-60+	12.5	Heriot et al[35]
Islands of Bougainville and Malaita, Solomon Islands	Nasioi and Kwaio tribes (rural)	512	0-89	0.3	Verlee[36]
Singapore	Malaysian (urban)	3280	40-79	12.3* (7.1-22.0)	Cajucom-Uy et al[29]
Sumatra, Indonesia	Malay-Indonesian (rural)	1210	21+	10.0* (2.9-17.3)	Gazzard et al[30]
Pulau Jaloh, Riau Archipelago, Indonesia	Indonesian (rural)	447	0-90	17 (1.9-56.0)	Tan et al[37]
Meiktila District, Central Myanmar	Burman (rural)	2076	40+	19.6 (14.0-21.6)	Durkin et al[38]
Tanjong Pagar district, Singapore	Chinese (urban)	1232	40-81	6.9* (2.2-15.3)	Wong et al[39]
Doumen County, China	Chinese (rural)	4214	50+	33.1	Wu et al[40]
Beijing, China	Chinese (rural and urban)	4439	40+	2.88 (1.13-5.84)	Ma et al[41]
Zeku County, China	Tibetan (rural and urban)	2229	40-80+	14.49 (10.1-24.2)	Lu et al[42]
Henan County, China	Mongolian (rural)	2112	40-80+	17.8* (13.5-27.5)	Lu et al[43]
Kumejima Island, Japan	Japanese (rural)	3747	40-80+	30.8	Shiroma et al[44]

Korea
  Buan-Kun, Chunbuk
  Dobong-Ku, Seoul
	
	Korean (rural)
	Korean (urban)
		
		686
		997
			0-70+	
				13.0
				3.5
					Kim et al[45]

Punjab, Parkistan	Pakistani	511	0-70+	26**	Hussain et al[46]
Tehran	Persian Turkish Kurd Arab Other	3673 727 62 14 69	1-60+	0.9 2.7 3.6 0 5.3	Fotouhi et al[47]
Copenhagen, Denmark	Caucasians	810	0-80+	0.7	Norn[48]

(continued)

TABLE 1-1. GLOBAL PREVALENCE OF PTERYGIA BY GEOGRAPHIC LOCATION (POPULATION-BASED SURVEYS ONLY) (continued)

GEOGRAPHIC LOCATION	POPULATION GROUP	SAMPLE SIZE	AGE (YEARS)	% PREVALENCE OVERALL (RANGE)	STUDY
Greenland	Eskimos	659	0-80+	8.6	Norn[48]
Tindouf, Algeria	Berber/Arabs	1322	2-87	18.0	Bueno-Gimeno et al[49]
Anambra, Nigeria	Nigerian (rural)	510	18-49	8.2	Nwosu[50]
Calvinia, Karoo, Cape Province	Colored (no details)	1660	0-70+	5.72	Hill[51]
Barbados, West Indies	Black Mixed White	2617 97 67	40-84	23.4 23.7 10.2	Luthra et al[52]
Arizona, USA	Hispanic	4774	40-80+	16.2 (13.7-19.1)	West & Munoz[53]
Amazon, Brazil	Arawak Tukanom Maku Yanomami	160 105 43 316	Adults	36.3 37.1 2.3 5.4	Paula et al[54]

* Age adjusted value.
** Pterygium and pinguecula were combined in this study.

Pathogenic Theories and Molecular Mechanisms

The pathogenesis of pterygium remains poorly understood and a subject of continued research. Our current understanding is that multiple processes are involved and these may be divided into inherited factors, environmental triggers (UV light, viral infections), and factors that perpetuate its growth (cytokines, GFs, and MMPs). In the following chapter, we will outline the theories and mechanisms on its pathogenesis.

UV light

Chronic UV exposure is the single most significant factor in the pathogenesis of pterygium. The relationship between UV exposure and pterygia is well supported by epidemiological studies,[9,22,55] and its association with other UV-related conditions such as photoaged skin,[10] cataracts,[56] climatic droplet keratopathy,[55] and squamous cell and basal cell carcinomas.[7,57] Pterygium frequently occurs at the medial limbus, which has been predicted by a ray tracing model to receive the maximal dose of UV light (Figure 1-4).[2,58] More recently, we have demonstrated UV-induced fluorescence at the nasal limbus (Figure 1-5)[59] in otherwise clinically normal school children.[60] These changes may represent the earliest evidence of solar-induced damage of the ocular surface.

Pterygia share certain histological features with photoaged skin such as epidermal proliferation, inflammatory infiltrates, activated fibroblasts, accumulation of elastin, glycosaminoglycans, and ECM remodeling.[61-65] To follow, we will illustrate

Figure 1-4. Light focusing effect of the anterior chamber. Incidental light is concentrated by the anterior chamber 20-fold onto the limbus where corneal stem cells reside. Chronic UV damage is hypothesized to alter limbal stem cells, leading to the formation of a pterygium.

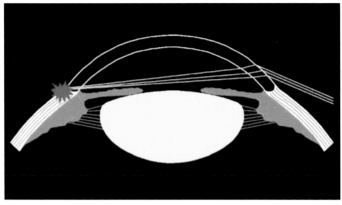

Figure 1-5. Solar exposure induced auto-fluorescence in a pterygium. A small pterygium photographed under (A) visible light and (B) UV light. Fluorescence is demonstrated at the advancing head of the pterygium. It has been speculated that fluorescent areas represent altered ECM components or abnormal cellular proliferation.

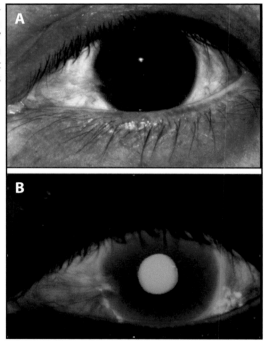

UV-activated molecular mechanisms such as oxidative stress and GF receptor (GFR) signaling that leads to synthesis and secretion of effector molecules such as cytokines, GFs, and MMPs that perpetuate the growth of pterygia (Figure 1-6).

Oxidative Stress and Growth Factor Receptor Signaling

Reactive oxygen species (ROS) are generated as a byproduct of metabolism and they react chemically with cellular components, leading to deoxyribonucleic acid (DNA) damage, lipid peroxidation, and alterations to protein structure and function. Endogenous antioxidants counteract the effect of ROS, and oxidative stress occurs when this process becomes overwhelmed.[66,67] UV is a well-known inducer of oxidative stress and a contributor to cutaneous photoaging.[68] Similar processes occur on the ocular surface in aging corneas, which are more susceptible to oxidative stress due to a reduction in antioxidants,[69] and repeated UV exposure further contributes to this problem.[66]

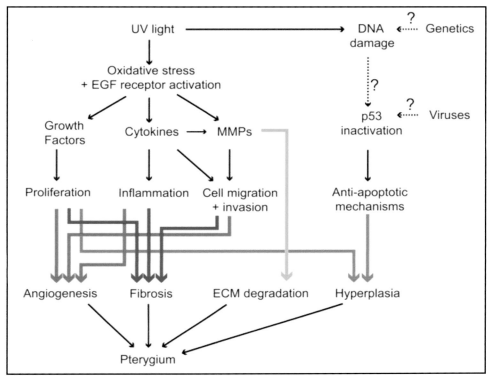

Figure 1-6. UV light activates multiple processes that may contribute to the formation of a pterygium. UV induces oxidative stress and epidermal GFR activation, leading to production of cytokines, GFs, and MMPs. These effector molecules mediate influx of inflammatory cells, angiogenesis, proliferation, fibrosis, and ECM degradation commonly observed in pterygia.

Oxidative stress is implicated in the pathogenesis of pterygia and other ocular conditions such as age-related cataract, keratoconus, and glaucoma.[70-74] Evidence for oxidative stress in pterygium includes the presence of 8-OHdG (a DNA photo-oxidation product)[75-77] and malondialdehyde (a product of lipid peroxidation),[78,79] inducible nitric oxide synthase (iNOS) and nitric oxide (NO),[80] and a reduction of antioxidants[81] in pterygium tissue. ROS species such as NO may act as a pro-angiogenic factor by mediating vascular sprouting,[82] endothelial proliferation, and migration.[45] NO promotes MMP-2 activity and reduces tissue inhibitors of metalloproteinase (TIMP-1) expression in corneal fibroblasts,[83] and similar mechanisms may account for MMP expression patterns in pterygia.[6] Other ROS such as hydrogen peroxide mediates UV-induced activation of epidermal GFRs (EGFRs) and subsequent downstream signaling via the mitogen activated protein kinase pathways.[84,85] These pathways are partially responsible for expression of proinflammatory cytokines[86] and MMPs[87,88] in pterygium cells.

Cytokines, Growth Factors, and Matrix Metalloproteinases

Cytokines, GFs, and MMPs serve physiological roles during corneal wound-healing[89-91] and have been implicated in the pathogenesis of pterygium.[6] UV exposure is reported to induce proinflammatory cytokines (interleukin 1 [IL-1], IL-6, IL-8, tumor necrosis factor alpha [TNF-α]); GFs (fibroblast GF 2 [FGF-2], vascular endothelial GF [VEGF], heparin-binding epidermal GF [HB-EGF], transforming GF alpha [TGF-α], stem

TABLE 1-2. CYTOKINES AND PROINFLAMMATORY MEDIATORS IN PTERYGIA

PROTEIN	FUNCTIONAL ROLE IN PTERYGIA	REFERENCES
CD30	Cell proliferation	142
COX-2	Prostaglandin synthesis, proinflammatory, antiapoptotic	117,118,119
Defensins, α1 and α2	Immune response, antimicrobial defense	124
Erythropoietin receptor	Cytokine receptor, proliferation, pro-angiogenic	143
IL-1	Cytokine, proinflammatory, pro-angiogenic, pro-fibrotic	114
IL-4	Cytokine, Th2 phenotype, pro-fibrotic	115
IL-6	Cytokine, proinflammatory	94
IL-8	Cytokine, chemoattractant, proinflammatory, pro-angiogenic	94
TNF-α	Cytokine, inflammation, pro-fibrotic, pro-angiogenic	113,144
SCF	Proinflammatory, mast cell maturation	128
S100 calcium-binding protein A6 (S100A6)	Cell proliferation	123
S100A8	Proinflammatory	123,124
S100A9	Proinflammatory	123,124,145

cell factor [SCF])[92-99]; and MMP-1.[87] These effector molecules contribute to inflammation, proliferation, angiogenesis, fibrosis, and ECM changes reported in pterygium.[6] Studies that investigated the role these molecules play in the pathogenesis of pterygium are listed in Tables 1-2 and 1-3. Though it is beyond the scope of this book to discuss each in detail, we will consider them in functional groups.

Cytokines, Proinflammatory Mediators, and Immunological Mechanisms

Chronic inflammation induced by desiccation,[100,101] chemical exposure,[102] antigens from solar radiation denatured proteins,[103] microtrauma,[104] or irritation from hairs on the caruncle or inner canthus[105] were previously hypothesized to contribute to the pathogenesis of pterygium. Wong suggested a mechanism where inflammation at the junction of the conjunctival blood vessels and Bowman's membrane degraded proteins, which then act as angiogenic factors.[106] Immunological mechanisms[107,108] might play a role given the presence of T-lymphocytes, plasma cells, mast cells, Langerhans cells, monocytes, macrophages,[107-111] immunoglobulins (IgG and IgE),[107,108] aberrant human leukocyte antigen (HLA-DR) expression by pterygium epithelium,[110] and elevated inter- and vascular cellular adhesion molecules (ICAM-1 and VCAM-1).[112] Although immune infiltrates may contribute to inflammation in pterygia, their presence are likely a consequence of cytokines and other proinflammatory mediators present in these ocular lesions.[6]

Classic UV-induced proinflammatory cytokines such as interleukins (IL-1, IL-6, IL-8), and TNF-α mediate an influx of immune cells and induce MMP expression in pterygia,[94,113,114] while IL-4 may mediate fibrosis in recurrent lesions.[115] Cyclooxygenase-2 (COX-2), a UV inducible enzyme that converts arachidonic acid into prostaglandins,[116] is overexpressed pterygia,[117,118] and its expression is associated with the antiapoptotic factor survivin.[119] COX-2 induces MMP-1 and MMP-9 in organ cultured corneas[120] and may also contribute to elevated MMP expression in pterygia. S100 proteins are calcium-binding proteins that have roles in wound healing, inflammation, and cancer[121,122] and have recently been described to be elevated in pterygium tissue[123] and in the tears of patients

TABLE 1-3. GROWTH FACTORS, THEIR RECEPTORS, AND RELATED PROTEINS IN PTERYGIA

GROWTH FACTORS	RECEPTORS	FUNCTIONAL ROLES IN PTERYGIA	REFERENCES
EGF; HB-EGF	EGFR; ErbB2; ErbB3	Mitogen; pro-fibrotic; pro-angiogenic	88, 95, 146-148
FGF-2	FGFR-1	Mitogen; pro-fibrotic; pro-angiogenic	113, 131, 144, 149
NGF; CNTF; NT4	TrkA; NGFR	Mitogen; pro-angiogenic	150-152
PDGF	PDGFR-β	Mitogen; pro-fibrotic; pro-angiogenic	113, 149
TGF-β	TGF-βRI; TGF-βRII; TGF-βRIII	Pro-fibrotic; pro-angiogenic	113, 144, 149, 153
VEGF	VEGFR1; VEGFR2	Pro-angiogenic	80, 154-158

PROTEINS	FUNCTIONAL ROLES IN PTERYGIA	REFERENCES
CTGF (IGFBP8)	Pro-fibrotic; pro-angiogenic	157
IGFBP2	Pro-fibrotic	159
IGFBP3	Anti-proliferative factor (decreased in pterygium)	160
PEDF	Angiogenic inhibitor (decreased in pterygium)	154, 161
THBS1	Angiogenic inhibitor (decreased in pterygium)	155

Abbreviations: EGF: epidermal growth factor; HBEGF: heparin-binding EGF-like growth factor; EGFR: epidermal growth factor receptor; ErbB: v-erb-b2 erythroblastic leukemia viral oncogene homolog; FGF-2: fibroblast growth factor-2; FGFR-1: fibroblast growth factor receptor-1; NGF: nerve growth factor; CNTF: ciliary neurotrophic factor; NT4: neurotrophin 4; TrkA: tyrosine kinase receptor A; NGFR: nerve growth factor receptor; PDGF: platelet-derived growth factor; PDGFR: platelet-derived growth factor receptor; TGF-β: transforming growth factor-β; TGF-βR: transforming growth factor-β receptor; VEGF: vascular endothelial growth factor; VEGFR: vascular endothelial growth factor receptor; CTGF: connective tissue growth factor; IGFBP: insulin-like growth factor binding protein; PEDF: pigment epithelium derived factor; THBS1: thrombospondin-1.

with pterygia.[124] The functional significance of S100 proteins in pterygia requires further study. However, their up-regulation may reflect induction by UV, cytokines, or other environmental stressors.[125-127] SCF is also elevated in the plasma and ocular tissues of patients with pterygia.[128,129] SCF attracts and induces maturation of mast cells, contributing to their elevated numbers in pterygium,[128,130] and their presence may promote fibrosis and neovascularization in pterygium.[131,132] Langerhans cells have also been observed in pterygium tissue by immunohistochemical[111] and in-vivo confocal studies.[133-135] It is speculated that a higher level of antigenic and mitogenic exposure[111] or the presence of cytokines in pterygium might have aided in their recruitment and maturation.[134] Their role in pterygium pathogenesis requires further study, but it suggests that Langerhans cells may be involved in T-cell recruitment in pterygium.[136]

It is interesting to note that while clinical evidence supports the notion that persistent inflammation may lead to postoperative recurrence,[137] this may be reduced by immunomodulators such as topical cyclosporine.[138,139] The quantity of infiltrating T-cells in pterygium specimens did not correlate with clinical parameters such as severity of inflammation, preoperative use of topical steroids, or non-steroidal anti-inflammatory drugs,[140] nor could recurrence be predicted by histological appearance.[141] This implies that inflammation does not act alone and that other factors may also contribute to recurrence of a pterygium.

Growth Factors and Their Receptors

GFs and their receptors have been described in pterygia (see Table 1-3). These molecules induce proliferation and/or migration of epithelial cells, fibroblasts, or vascular cells, processes that contribute to hyperplasia, fibrosis, and angiogenesis in pterygium.[4,6]

Pro-fibrotic cytokines and GFs expressed in pterygia include IL-1, TNF-α, connective tissue GF (CTGF), EGF family, FGF-2, platelet-derived GF (PDGF), and TGF-β.[4] Of these, TGF-β is particularly important since it induces myofibroblast differentiation and epithelial mesenchymal transition (EMT) and alters synthesis of ECM components.[90,162] Aberrant TGF-β signaling[113,144] is thought to contribute to fibrosis in pterygia and its suppression by amniotic membrane[149] may explain the efficacy of this treatment.

Elevated pro-angiogenic factors (IL-8, TNF-α, FGF-2, HB-EGF, and VEGF)[80,94,95,113] combined with lack of angiogenic inhibitors (pigment epithelium-derived factor [PEDF] and thrombospondin-1)[154,155] encourage prominent neovascularization in pterygia.[156,163] VEGF, a major pro-angiogenic factor, is elevated in the tears, plasma, and ocular tissues of patients with pterygia.[80,129,154,155] VEGF expression in pterygium may be driven by multiple stimuli (UV, hypoxia, cytokines, and GFs),[86,129,164,165] and probably represent a common pro-angiogenic pathway. Therefore, VEGF inhibition is currently under investigation as a treatment for this condition.[166,167]

More recently, neurotrophins and their receptors have been investigated in pterygia, where nerve GF (NGF), ciliary neurotrophic factor (CNTF), and neurotrophin-4/5 were reported to be elevated. In addition, the high and low affinity NGF receptors (tyrosine kinase receptor A [TRKA] and NGFR, respectively) have also been described in pterygium epithelial cells and blood vessels.[150-152] A pro-angiogenic role for neurotrophins is suggested by the correlation of NGF-TRKA staining with microvessel density in pterygia.[151]

Matrix Metalloproteinases and Extracellular Matrix Remodeling

For many years, pterygia were considered degenerative in nature due to prominent ECM changes. This concept likely originated from the term *elastotic degeneration* used to describe worm-like fibers in the subepithelial tissues that took on elastic stain but were considered to be altered collagen due to their resistance to elastase digestion.[168,169] Reinforcing the theme of degeneration is dissolution of Bowman's layer at the advancing head of the pterygium,[170,171] which is now attributed to the action of MMPs.[6,172] In fact, both abnormal synthesis and breakdown of matrix components occur in pterygia, and even Duke-Elder acknowledged that pterygium is a degenerative and hyperplastic condition.[171]

MMPs are a family of zinc-dependent endopeptidases that degrade components of the ECM and cell surface molecules.[91] MMPs may be secreted or membrane bound, and their actions are counterbalanced by tissue inhibitors of metalloproteinases (TIMPs). MMPs play roles in ocular physiology and pathophysiology and are key mediators of photoaging, in which they regulate proliferation, cell migration, inflammation, and angiogenesis.[91,173,174] Epithelium, fibroblasts, vascular cells, and infiltrating immune cells have been reported to produce MMPs in pterygia.[172,175-179] Overexpression of MMPs relative to TIMPs at the head of the pterygium is thought to contribute to the invasive phenotype of this condition.[172,175] UV exposure, cytokines (IL-1 and TNF-α), and GFs (EGF and TGF-α) have all been shown to induce expression of MMPs in pterygium cells.[87,175,176,180] Furthermore, MMP-2 and MMP-9 are associated with disease progression,[181] suggesting that MMPs may be an attractive target for management of this disease.

In addition to ECM breakdown, altered synthesis of matrix components have been reported in pterygium, including abnormal tropoelastin,[182] glycosaminoglycans,[183] hyaluronic acid,[184] and periostin.[115] Altered matrix components may increase the bioavailability of HB-EGFs and cytokines (eg, IL-8, FGF-2, HB-EGF, VEGF, PDGF, and TGF-β), which are normally sequestered by the ECM and released upon degradation of the ECM.[185,186]

Pterygium as a Disease of Stem Cells

Epithelial Stem Cells

The limbus is a transitional zone separating the transparent cornea from the vascularized conjunctiva. This specialized region, called the *limbal niche*, harbors stem cells that retain the ability to divide and repopulate the ocular surface throughout an individual's lifetime.[187,188] Chronic UV exposure is hypothesized to alter limbal stem cells and take on an infiltrative phenotype, giving rise to a pterygium.[2,189] The stem cell origins of pterygia are supported by shared biomarkers between pterygium and limbal epithelium such as cytokeratins[189,190]; vimentin[189]; telomerase[191,192]; tumor protein p63[87,193-195]; ATP-binding cassette, sub-family G, member 2 (ABCG2)[152]; and NGFR.[152] Conversely, pterygium also has features suggestive of limbal stem cell deficiency, such as an absence of normal limbal palisades (Figure 1-7), ingrowth of conjunctival-like epithelium,[196,197] and vascularization of the cornea.[163,198,199] Further supporting this notion is the fact that restoration of stem cell populations via autologous limbal grafts has been reported to be an effective treatment for both primary and recurrent pterygia.[200,201]

Epithelial Mesenchymal Transition

EMT, a process by which epithelial cells take on characteristics of mesenchymal cells, has been described in pterygia[190,202] and may provide an explanation for the origin of pterygium fibroblasts. Kato and colleagues[190] described changes in pterygium that resembled EMT. They reported pterygium cells co-expressing an epithelial marker (cytokeratin 14) with mesenchymal markers (α-smooth muscle actin and vimentin) extending toward the pterygium stroma, and noted the presence of signaling molecules associated with EMT (nuclear localization of β-catenin, snail, and slug).[190] Their findings imply that pterygium fibroblasts might have originated from limbal epithelium through EMT and the presence of GFs such as TGF-β[203] and FGF-2,[204] or UV exposure[205] may mediate this process. An alternate theory is that pterygium fibroblasts may be recruited from myofibroblasts in the periorbital fibroadipose tissue posterior to Tenon's capsule since they share similar immunohistological characteristics of α-smooth muscle actin staining and did not stain for desmin or caldesmon.[206]

Bone Marrow-Derived Progenitor Cells

Bone marrow-derived progenitor cells expressing hematopoietic (CD34, AC133, or c-kit positive) or mesenchymal (STRO-1 positive) markers have been reported in pterygium and are hypothesized to contribute to the fibrovascular stroma.[207,208] Supporting this concept is the presence of bone marrow-derived cells in the normal corneal stroma[209] together with animal models showing recruitment of bone marrow-derived cells to areas of active fibrosis[210] and neovascularization.[211] Ocular tissue hypoxia-induced cytokines are thought to act as chemoattractants to the eye[211] and in pterygia. Lee et al showed that patients with pterygia had elevated circulating CD34 and c-kit positive progenitor cells as well as plasma VEGF, SCF, and Substance P (SP).[129]

Figure 1-7. Confocal examination of the normal corneal limbus and a pterygium. Normal limbal structures potentially damaged by chronic UV exposure include (A) the palisades of Vogt and (B) perilimbal nerves. In pterygium, abnormal limbal architecture is demonstrated at (C) the head of a pterygium, whilst fibroblastic proliferation is present in (D) the pterygium stroma.

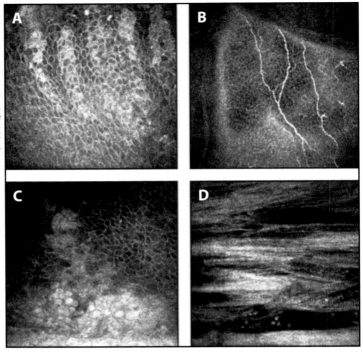

Abnormal Proliferation and Antiapoptotic Mechanisms

Pterygia are often considered as benign tumors due to their invasive growth habit and propensity for recurrence but not metastasis. The notion that pterygia may be pre-neoplastic was initially suggested by Sevel and Sealy, who observed that 29% of pterygia had dysplastic changes.[212] Since then, others have also reported concurrent pre-neoplastic diseases such as ocular surface squamous neoplasia (~10%)[213] and primary acquired melanosis (~9%).[214]

Abnormal proliferation has been documented in pterygium epithelium and stroma. Specifically, antiapoptotic proteins (BCL-2[215] and survivin[119]) and cell proliferation-associated molecules (cyclin D1, Ki67, and proliferating cell nuclear antigen)[216-218] were shown to be elevated in pterygium epithelial cells, and increased DNA content reported in the fibrovascular layer.[219] In addition, pterygium fibroblast cultures exhibit other features associated with a transformed phenotype, such as reduced serum dependence and anchorage independent growth,[220] altered lipid metabolism,[221] and expression of insulin-like GF-binding proteins, which are also known to be altered in cancers.[159,160,222]

Inherited Factors

Although the presence of pterygia is strongly associated with environmental exposure, inherited factors may also play a role in its development. There are reports of families or close relatives with pterygia, and in these cases, ocular lesions often present at an early age.[223-226] An inheritance pattern of autosomal dominant with incomplete penetrance has also been reported.[227,228] Hereditary defects in DNA repair may account for a high incidence of bilateral pterygia in patients with xeroderma pigmentosum.[229] Genetic association studies suggest that single nucleotide polymorphisms (SNPs) or

TABLE 1-4. GENETIC ASSOCIATION STUDIES ON PATIENTS WITH PTERYGIA

GENE	FUNCTION	GENETIC VARIANT	DBSNP ACCESSION NUMBER	ASSOCIATION WITH PTERYGIUM
OGG1	DNA repair	Exon 7, 1245C>G	rs1052133	Yes[230]
GSTM1	DNA repair	Gene deletion, Null genotype	–	Yes[231]
XRCC6	DNA repair	Promoter, -991C>T	rs5751129	Yes[232]
		Promoter, -57G>C	rs2267437	No[232]
TP53	Tumor suppressor, DNA repair	Exon 4, 119C>G	rs1042522	No[233-235]
CDKN1A	Cell cycle regulator, DNA repair	Exon 2, 98C>A	rs1801270	No[233]
TNF	Inflammation	Promoter, -308G>A	rs1800629	No[236]
IL1B	Inflammation	Promoter, -511C>T	rs16944	No[236]
		Exon 5, +3954C>T	rs1143634	No[236]
IL1RN	Inflammation (antagonist)	Intron 2, VNTR of 86bp, Alleles 1, 2, 3, 4 and 5	–	No[236]
VEGFA	Angiogenesis	Promoter, -460T>C	rs833061	Yes,[237] No[238]
TGFB1	Cytokine, proliferation, differentiation, fibrosis	Promoter, -509C>T	rs1800469	No[238]

Abbreviations: OGG1: 8-oxoguanine DNA glycosylase; GSTM1: glutathione S-transferase M1; XRCC6: x-ray repair complementing defective repair in Chinese hamster cells 6; TP53: tumor suppressor p53 protein; CDKN1A: cyclin-dependent kinase inhibitor 1A; TNF: tumor necrosis factor-α; IL1B: interleukin-1β; IL1RN: interleukin-1 receptor antagonist; VEGFA: vascular endothelial growth factor; TGFB1: transforming growth factor-β1; VNTR: variable number tandem repeat.

With the exception of one study on Brazilians,[235] all studies were performed on the Taiwanese population.

other genetic variants in the 8-oxoguanine glycosylase (OGG1), glutathione S-transferase Mu 1 (GSTM1), and X-ray repair complementing defective repair in Chinese hamster cells 6 (XRCC6) genes may contribute to the pathogenesis of pterygia (Table 1-4). However, current reports remain limited to small, single population studies and should be interpreted with caution.

Deoxyribonucleic Acid Damage and Tumor Suppressor

A number of genetic changes have been described in pterygia, including loss of heterozygosity and microsatellite instability,[239] point mutations in the Kirsten-*ras* gene,[240] mutations of the p53 gene,[241-243] and hypermethylation of the p16 promoter.[244] Of these, only p53 mutations have been studied extensively. p53 is a tumor suppressor protein normally found in low levels in the cytoplasm due to its short half-life. In the presence of DNA damage, it stabilizes; translocates to the nucleus; and induces cell cycle arrest, DNA repair, or apoptosis.[245] Normal p53 function prevents accumulation of genetic aberrations, and UV-induced mutations of p53 are frequently present in skin cancers.[246] Dushku and Reid proposed that inactivating mutations of p53 contributed to the pathogenesis of pterygium by impairment of the p53-dependent programmed cell death mechanism, allowing gene mutations to accumulate and leading to the formation of pterygia.[247] They observed by immunohistochemical methods that nuclear expression of p53 was elevated in pterygia without concurrent apoptosis.[247] Since then, others have also reported elevated p53 staining in pterygia relative to normal conjunctival tissues,[215,217,248-251] yet p53 staining did not correlate with recurrence,[249,250] and some pterygia did not stain for p53.[252] Using the gold standard method of DNA sequencing, it was found that the p53 gene had undergone monoallelic deletion (4 of 9 cases)[243] or point mutations (8 out of 51 cases).[241] Furthermore, accumulation of p53 protein may not necessarily be accompanied by mutations of the p53 gene[253] and deletion mutations may lead to loss of p53 expression.[232] To confound these findings even further, one report suggests an alternate mechanism for inactivation of p53 by viral oncoprotein (human papillomavirus [HPV] 16/18 E6).[242] Therefore, more DNA sequencing studies are required to establish the prevalence of p53 mutations and their role in the pathogenesis of pterygia.

Viral Infections

A role for viruses in the pathogenesis of pterygia was suggested by Detorakis et al, where they proposed a "2-hit" hypothesis.[254] The first hit is attributed to a genetic predisposition for pterygia or acquired DNA damage from UV exposure. The second hit may be additional UV exposure or infections of HPV or herpes simplex virus (HSV).

Supporting a viral etiology in the pathogenesis of pterygium is the detection of HPV DNA in 3% to 100% of pterygia (Table 1-5). This variation may be explained by different methods employed by investigators to detect HPV, or alternatively explained by variable HPV infection rates between population groups.[255] One study also suggests that viral oncoprotein (HPV 16/18 E6) may inactivate p53.[242] However, current opinion is that HPV is not an absolute requirement for pterygium development given that positive HPV rates were low to undetectable in some studies.[256-259]

Studies on HSV and pterygia are currently limited to 2 centers. In Greece, 11/50 pterygia cases (22%) were HSV-positive and 3/50 pterygia cases (6%) were coinfected with HPV and may be associated with postoperative recurrence.[260] In Taiwan, 3/65 pterygia cases (5%) were HSV-positive and all lesions were primary, although recurrent samples were negative.[261] A role for HSV in the pathogenesis of pterygia remains unclear given a lack of evidence. Without an in-vivo model of pterygia formation, it remains difficult to prove or disprove a causal role of viral infections in the development of pterygia.

Neurogenic Model

The above theories do not explain some aspects of pterygia, such as its centripetal growth pattern that gives rise to its characteristic wing-like appearance. To address this issue, a neurogenic model was proposed, whereby corneal nerves may influence the centripetal migration of corneal epithelium and pterygium cells.[4,262] This model is based on several observations:

- Normal corneal epithelial turnover as summarized in the XYZ hypothesis,[263] which shows our previously postulated cell population balanced model[58] that may in part explain the wing shape of pterygium

- The radial arrangement of corneal nerves and their close relationship with corneal epithelium and keratocytes[264]

- Involvement of sensory neurons in wound healing and inflammation[265-268]

- The presence of myelinated and unmyelinated nerve fibers within the connective tissue mass of pterygia[269,270]

TABLE 1-5. POLYMERASE CHAIN REACTION DETECTION OF HUMAN PAPILLOMAVIRUS IN PTERYGIA

INVESTIGATORS (COUNTRY)	SAMPLE TYPES	POSITIVE RATE (%)	HPV SUBTYPES
Dushku et al (United States)[257]	13 pterygia	0	Nil detected
Gallagher et al (United Kingdom)[271]	10 pterygia	50	6, 11, 16
Detorakis et al (Greece)[260]	50 pterygia	24	18
Piras et al (Italy)[255]	17 pterygia	100	52, 54, candHPV90
Piras et al (Ecuador)[255]	24 pterygia	21	52, 54, candHPV90
Chen et al (Taiwan)[256]	65 primary pterygia	0	Nil detected
Schellini et al (Brazil)[258]	36 primary pterygia	0	Nil detected
Sjo et al (Denmark)[272]	100 primary pterygia	4.4	6
Takamura et al (Japan)[273]	42 pterygia	4.8	Not tested
Rodrigues et al (Brazil)[235]	36 pterygia	58.3	1, 2
Guthoff et al (Germany)[259]	11 pterygia	0	Nil detected
Otlu et al (Turkey)[274]	40 pterygia (30 primary, 10 recurrent)	0	Nil detected
Piecyk-Sidor et al (Poland)[275]	58 pterygia	27.6	6, 16, 18
Tsai et al (Taiwan)[242]	129 pterygia	24	16, 18
Hsiao et al (Taiwan)[276]	65 pterygia (35 primary, 30 recurrent)	3	18

The limbus is the focal point of chronic UV exposure,[3] where limbal epithelium, stromal cells, blood vessels, and the perilimbal nerve plexus[277,278] may be subject to UV damage (Figure 1-8). While studies of ocular responses to UV light focused on epithelium and stromal cells, the neuronal response to UV injury may also be an important trigger for the development of pterygia since the normal cornea is a highly innervated structure.[264] UV exposure may induce release of sensory neuropeptides, such as SP and calcitonin gene-related peptide (CGRP), which participate in neurogenic inflammation through their roles as vasodilators and immune cell chemoattractant, and by inducing cytokine production from resident corneal cells to amplify the inflammatory response.[145,154,165,166] SP and CGRP may also induce proliferation and migration of corneal epithelial cells[146,150-152,167] and fibroblasts,[147,148,153,157] and may contribute to angiogenesis.[45,158] In pterygium, SP and its receptor (NK1R) are expressed by epithelial cells, fibroblasts, and infiltrating immune cells and have been shown to induce migration of pterygium fibroblasts and vascular endothelium, suggesting a pro-fibroangiogenic role.[262] The above evidence together with the distribution of corneal nerves[264] suggests that corneal nerves might play a role in the development of pterygia.

Predictors or Biomarkers for Recurrence

A central problem in the surgical management of pterygium is the rate of recurrence. While some factors contributing to recurrences have been identified, the process remains poorly understood. To date, predictors or biomarkers for recurrence are not

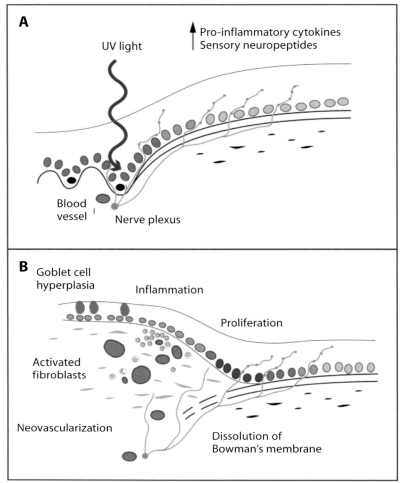

Figure 1-8. A neurogenic model for the pathogenesis of pterygium. UV light damages the perilimbal nerve plexus, blood vessels, as well as stem cells residing in the limbal niche. (A) Injured corneal nerves release sensory neuropeptides such as SP and CGRP, leading to production of proinflammatory cytokines and chemokines. (B) In the later stage, corneal nerves may act as a scaffold for migrating fibroblasts and vascular endothelial cells.

well defined for pterygia. Many variables may contribute to the recurrence of a lesion and these may be related to the patient (genetics, environmental exposure, the nature of the lesion) or the surgeon (treatment methods, clinical experience). Few studies are able to address all of these factors, and this area requires further research.

Clinical Predictors of Recurrence

Tan et al described a pterygia grading system based on the visibility of episcleral vessels as an indicator of the thickness of the lesion.[279] Pterygia were categorized into atrophic (T1, visible episcleral vessels), intermediate (T2, partially obscured episcleral vessels), or fleshy (T3, obscured episcleral vessels) and it was shown that nontranslucency (or fleshiness) was a significant risk factor for recurrence in patients managed by bare scleral excision.[279]

Racial factors may also influence recurrence rates. One study reports higher recurrences rates in Hispanics than in Whites.[280] However, the confounding factor of lifestyle (ie, sun exposure) may be different in these patient groups.

Biomarkers of Recurrence

The recurrence of a pterygium could not be predicted by histological and immunohistological parameters such as vascularization, morphological signs of dry eye, or reactive inflammation.[141] However, recurrent pterygia are reported to have several biological characteristics. Loss of heterozygosity at 9q31-33 is more frequent.[281] Significantly elevated DNA content has been reported in the fibrovascular layer,[219] and recurrent pterygium fibroblast cultures migrate and proliferate faster than those from primary pterygia.[282] Full thickness staining of p63 and p16 pterygium epithelium was reported in recurrent pterygia,[283] which may reflect an increase in epithelial cell proliferation. Pro-angiogenic GFs such as VEGF and SP are elevated in the tears and plasma of patients with recurrence.[129] Genome-wide expression studies comparing primary with recurrent pterygia have identified several markers that are associated with recurrence. These include periostin, TIMP-2, L-3-phosphoserine phosphatase homolog (PSPHL), sialophorin (SPN) and never in mitosis a-5 (NEK), with roles in cell adhesion and motility.[284,285]

These biomarkers for recurrence require further evaluation to assess their clinical predictive value. They also imply that treatment strategies for pterygium should target multiple pathways (proliferation, inflammation, fibrosis, and angiogenesis) in order to be successful.

Conclusion

Research of the enigmatic pterygium has not only provided insight into the interaction of UV light with the ocular surface, but also how this knowledge may improve methods of managing this persistent condition. Rather than the historical view of pterygium as a degenerative condition, the complex, active processes of cell proliferation, hyperplasia, migration and invasion, inflammation, angiogenesis, fibrosis, and ECM degradation have been revealed. We now have a working model where UV-induced oxidative stress, GF signaling, cytokines, and MMPs mediate the growth of pterygia and Bowman's membrane destruction. The contribution of limbal and bone marrow stem cells have been explored, as well as the potential role of neurogenic inflammation from UV injured corneal nerves. Individual susceptibilities such as genetics and previous viral infections may also contribute to the DNA damage observed in some of these lesions. A number of biomarkers in recurrent pterygium have been identified but require further evaluation. Given the various mechanisms involved, medical interventions for pterygia may need to target multiple pathways that have been identified in its pathogenesis.

References

1. Coroneo MT, Muller-Stolzenburg NW, Ho A. Peripheral light focusing by the anterior eye and the ophthalmohelioses. *Ophthalmic Surg.* 1991;22(12):705-711.
2. Coroneo MT. Pterygium as an early indicator of ultraviolet insolation: a hypothesis. *Br J Ophthalmol.* 1993;77(11):734-739.
3. Coster D. Pterygium—an ophthalmic enigma. *Br J Ophthalmol.* 1995;79(4):304-305.

4.   Chui J, Di Girolamo N, Wakefield D, Coroneo MT. The pathogenesis of pterygium: current concepts and their thera-peutic implications. *Ocul Surf.* 2008;6(1):24-43.
5.   Coroneo MT, Di Girolamo N, Wakefield D. The pathogenesis of pterygia. *Curr Opin Ophthalmol.* 1999;10(4):282-288.
6.   Di Girolamo N, Chui J, Coroneo MT, Wakefield D. Pathogenesis of pterygia: role of cytokines, growth factors, and matrix metalloproteinases. *Prog Retin Eye Res.* 2004;23(2):195-228.
7.   Kerkenezov N. A pterygium survey of the far north coast of New South Wales. *Trans Ophthalmol Soc Aust.* 1956;16:110-119.
8.   Li M, Zhang M, Lin Y, et al. Tear function and goblet cell density after pterygium excision. *Eye.* 2007;21(2):224-228.
9.   Moran DJ, Hollows FC. Pterygium and ultraviolet radiation: a positive correlation. *Br J Ophthalmol.* 1984;68(5):343-346.
10.   Panchapakesan J, Hourihan F, Mitchell P. Prevalence of pterygium and pinguecula: the Blue Mountains Eye Study. *Aust N Z J Ophthalmol.* 1998;26(suppl 1):S2-5.
11.   Wlodarczyk J, Whyte P, Cockrum P, Taylor H. Pterygium in Australia: a cost of illness study. *Clin Experiment Ophthalmol.* 2001;29(6):370-375.
12.   Dolezalova V. Is the occurrence of a temporal pterygium really so rare? *Ophthalmologica.* 1977;174(2):88-91.
13.   Raizada IN, Bhatnagar NK. Pinguecula and pterygium (a histopathological study). *Indian J Ophthalmol.* 1976;24(2):16-18.
14.   Lemercier G, Cornand G, Burckhart MF. [Pinguecula and pterygium: histologic and electron microscopic study (author's transl)]. *Virchows Arch A Pathol Anat Histol.* 1978;379(4):321-333.
15.   Goldman KN, Kaufman HE. Atypical pterygium. A clinical feature of Terrien's marginal degeneration. *Arch Ophthalmol.* 1978;96(6):1027-1029.
16.   Gridley MJ, Perlman EM. A form of variable astigmatism induced by pseudopterygium. *Ophthalmic Surg.* 1986;17(12):794-795.
17.   Booth AJ, Hodgkins PR. Pseudopterygium arising in a patient with multiple keloids. *J Pediatr Ophthalmol Strabismus.* 2006;43(1):49-51.
18.   Gagnon MR, Dickinson PJ. Ocular surface injury from a microwave superheated egg resulting in a pseudopter-ygium. *Eye Contact Lens.* 2005;31(3):109-110.
19.   Gris O, Guell JL, del Campo Z. Limbal-conjunctival autograft transplantation for the treatment of recurrent pte-rygium. *Ophthalmology.* 2000;107(2):270-273.
20.   Wong AK, Rao SK, Leung AT, Poon AS, Lam DS. Inferior limbal-conjunctival autograft transplantation for recurrent pterygium. *Indian J Ophthalmol.* 2000;48(1):21-24.
21.   Wesley RE, Collins JW. Pseudopterygium from exposure to selenium dioxide. *Ann Ophthalmol.* 1982;14(6):588-589.
22.   Threlfall TJ, English DR. Sun exposure and pterygium of the eye: a dose-response curve. *Am J Ophthalmol.* 1999;128(3):280-287.
23.   Taylor HR, West SK, Rosenthal FS, Munoz B, Newland HS, Emmett EA. Corneal changes associated with chronic UV irradiation. *Arch Ophthalmol.* 1989;107(10):1481-1484.
24.   Mackenzie FD, Hirst LW, Battistutta D, Green A. Risk analysis in the development of pterygia. *Ophthalmology.* 1992;99(7):1056-1061.
25.   McCarty CA, Fu CL, Taylor HR. Epidemiology of pterygium in Victoria, Australia. *British Journal of Ophthalmology.* 2000;84(3):289-292.
26.   Wong TY, Foster PJ, Johnson GJ, Seah SK, Tan DT. The prevalence and risk factors for pterygium in an adult Chinese population in Singapore: the Tanjong Pagar survey. *American Journal of Ophthalmology.* 2001;131(2):176-183.
27.   Khoo J, Saw SM, Banerjee K, Chia SE, Tan D. Outdoor work and the risk of pterygia: a case-control study. *International Ophthalmology.* 1998;22(5):293-298.
28.   Lin W, Wang SL, Wu HJ, et al. Associations between arsenic in drinking water and pterygium in southwestern Taiwan. *Environ Health Perspect.* 2008;116(7):952-955.
29.   Cajucom-Uy HY, Tong LH, Wong TY, Tay WT, Saw SM. The prevalence of and risk factors for pterygium in an urban Malay population: the Singapore Malay Eye Study (SiMES). *Br J Ophthalmol.* 2010;94(8):977-981. Epub 2009 Dec 3.
30.   Gazzard G, Saw SM, Farook M, et al. Pterygium in Indonesia: prevalence, severity and risk factors. *Br J Ophthalmol.* 2002;86(12):1341-1346.
31.   Karai I, Horiguchi S. Pterygium in welders. *British Journal of Ophthalmology.* 1984;68(5):347-349.
32.   Nakaishi H, Yamamoto M, Ishida M, Someya I, Yamada Y. Pingueculae and pterygia in motorcycle policemen. *Industrial Health.* 1997;35(3):325-329.
33.   McCarty CA, Fu CL, Taylor HR. Epidemiology of pterygium in Victoria, Australia. *Br J Ophthalmol.* 2000;84(3):289-292.
34.   Mann I, Potter D. Geographic ophthalmology. A preliminary study of the Maoris of New Zealand. *Am J Ophthalmol.* 1969;67(3):358-369.
35.   Heriot WJ, Crock GW, Taylor R, Zimmet P. Ophthalmic findings among one thousand inhabitants of Rarotonga, Cook Islands. *Aust J Ophthalmol.* 1983;11(2):81-94.
36.   Verlee DL. Ophthalmic survey in the Solomon Islands. *Am J Ophthalmol.* 1968;66(2):304-319.
37.   Tan CS, Lim TH, Koh WP, et al. Epidemiology of pterygium on a tropical island in the Riau Archipelago. *Eye.* 2006;20(8):908-912.
38.   Durkin SR, Abhary S, Newland HS, Selva D, Aung T, Casson RJ. The prevalence, severity and risk factors for pte-rygium in central Myanmar: the Meiktila Eye Study. *Br J Ophthalmol.* 2008;92(1):25-29.

39. Wong TY, Foster PJ, Johnson GJ, Seah SK, Tan DT. The prevalence and risk factors for pterygium in an adult Chinese population in Singapore: the Tanjong Pagar survey. *Am J Ophthalmol.* 2001;131(2):176-183.
40. Wu K, He M, Xu J, Li S. Pterygium in aged population in Doumen County, China. *Yan Ke Xue Bao.* 2002;18(3):181-184.
41. Ma K, Xu L, Jie Y, Jonas JB. Prevalence of and factors associated with pterygium in adult Chinese: the Beijing Eye Study. *Cornea.* 2007;26(10):1184-1186.
42. Lu P, Chen X, Kang Y, Ke L, Wei X, Zhang W. Pterygium in Tibetans: a population-based study in China. *Clin Experiment Ophthalmol.* 2007;35(9):828-833.
43. Lu J, Wang Z, Lu P, et al. Pterygium in an aged Mongolian population: a population-based study in China. *Eye.* 2009;23(2):421-427.
44. Shiroma H, Higa A, Sawaguchi S, et al. Prevalence and risk factors of pterygium in a southwestern island of Japan: the Kumejima Study. *Am J Ophthalmol.* 2009;148(5):766-771, e761.
45. Kim WS, Kim IS, Hu JU, Kim JC, Kim JD, Koo BS. Community-based eye health survey in areas of Buan-Kun and Dobong-Ku in Korea. *Korean J Ophthalmol.* 1990;4(2):103-107.
46. Hussain A, Awan H, Khan MD. Prevalence of non-vision-impairing conditions in a village in Chakwal district, Punjab, Pakistan. *Ophthalmic Epidemiol.* 2004;11(5):413-426.
47. Fotouhi A, Hashemi H, Khabazkhoob M, Mohammad K. Prevalence and risk factors of pterygium and pinguecula: the Tehran Eye Study. *Eye.* 2009;23(5):1125-1129.
48. Norn MS. Spheroid degeneration of cornea and conjunctiva. Prevalence among Eskimos in Greenland and Caucasians in Copenhagen. *Acta Ophthalmol (Copenh).* 1978;56(4):551-562.
49. Bueno-Gimeno I, Montes-Mico R, Espana-Gregori E, Pons AM. Epidemiologic study of pterygium in a Saharan population. *Ann Ophthalmol.* 2002;34(1):43-46.
50. Nwosu SN. Ocular problems of young adults in rural Nigeria. *Int Ophthalmol.* 1998;22(5):259-263.
51. Hill JC. The prevalence of corneal disease in the coloured community of a Karoo town. *S Afr Med J.* 1985;67(18):723-727.
52. Luthra R, Nemesure BB, Wu SY, Xie SH, Leske MC. Frequency and risk factors for pterygium in the Barbados Eye Study. *Arch Ophthalmol.* 2001;119(12):1827-1832.
53. West S, Munoz B. Prevalence of pterygium in Latinos: Proyecto VER. *Br J Ophthalmol.* 2009;93(10):1287-1290.
54. Paula JS, Thorn F, Cruz AA. Prevalence of pterygium and cataract in indigenous populations of the Brazilian Amazon rain forest. *Eye.* 2006;20(5):533-536.
55. Taylor HR. Ultraviolet radiation and the eye: an epidemiologic study. *Trans Am Ophthalmol Soc.* 1989;87:802-853.
56. Lim R, Mitchell P, Cumming RG. Cataract associations with pinguecula and pterygium: the Blue Mountains Eye Study. *Am J Ophthalmol.* 1998;126(5):717-719.
57. Clear AS, Chirambo MC, Hutt MS. Solar keratosis, pterygium, and squamous cell carcinoma of the conjunctiva in Malawi. *Br J Ophthalmol.* 1979;63(2):102-109.
58. Kwok LS, Coroneo MT. A model for pterygium formation. *Cornea.* 1994;13(3):219-224.
59. Ooi JL, Sharma NS, Sharma S, et al. Ultraviolet fluorescence photography: patterns in established pterygia. *Am J Ophthalmol.* 2007;143(1):97-101.
60. Ooi JL, Sharma NS, Papalkar D, et al. Ultraviolet fluorescence photography to detect early sun damage in the eyes of school-aged children. *Am J Ophthalmol.* 2006;141(2):294-298.
61. Bielenberg DR, Bucana CD, Sanchez R, Donawho CK, Kripke ML, Fidler IJ. Molecular regulation of UVB-induced cutaneous angiogenesis. *J Invest Dermatol.* 1998;111(5):864-872.
62. Bissett DL, Hannon DP, Orr TV. An animal model of solar-aged skin: histological, physical, and visible changes in UV-irradiated hairless mouse skin. *Photochem Photobiol.* 1987;46(3): 367-378.
63. Fourtanier A, Berrebi C. Miniature pig as an animal model to study photoaging. *Photochem Photobiol.* 1989;50(6):771-784.
64. Koshiishi I, Horikoshi E, Mitani H, Imanari T. Quantitative alterations of hyaluronan and dermatan sulfate in the hairless mouse dorsal skin exposed to chronic UV irradiation. *Biochimica et Biophysica Acta.* 1999;1428(2-3):327-333.
65. Lee JH, An HT, Chung JH, Kim KH, Eun HC, Cho KH. Acute effects of UVB radiation on the proliferation and differentiation of keratinocytes. *Photodermatol Photoimmunol Photomed.* 2002;18(5):253-261.
66. Cejkova J, Stipek S, Crkovska J, Ardan T. Changes of superoxide dismutase, catalase and glutathione peroxidase in the corneal epithelium after UVB rays. Histochemical and biochemical study. *Histol Histopathol.* 2000;15(4):1043-1050.
67. Elahi MM, Naseem KM, Matata BM. Nitric oxide in blood. The nitrosative-oxidative disequilibrium hypothesis on the pathogenesis of cardiovascular disease. *Febs J.* 2007;274(4):906-923.
68. Wlaschek M, Tantcheva-Poor I, Naderi L, et al. Solar UV irradiation and dermal photoaging. *J Photochem Photobiol B.* 2001;63(1-3):41-51.
69. Cejkova J, Vejrazka M, Platenik J, Stipek S. Age-related changes in superoxide dismutase, glutathione per-oxidase, catalase and xanthine oxidoreductase/xanthine oxidase activities in the rabbit cornea. *Exp Gerontol.* 2004;39(10):1537-1543.
70. Truscott RJ. Age-related nuclear cataract-oxidation is the key. *Exp Eye Res.* 2005;80(5):709-725.
71. Algvere PV, Marshall J, Seregard S. Age-related maculopathy and the impact of blue light hazard. *Acta Ophthalmol Scand.* 2006;84(1):4-15.
72. Izzotti A, Bagnis A, Sacca SC. The role of oxidative stress in glaucoma. *Mutat Res.* 2006;612(2):105-114.
73. Buddi R, Lin B, Atilano SR, Zorapapel NC, Kenney MC, Brown DJ. Evidence of oxidative stress in human corneal diseases. *J Histochem Cytochem.* 2002;50(3):341-351.

74. Shoham A, Hadziahmetovic M, Dunaief JL, Mydlarski MB, Schipper HM. Oxidative stress in diseases of the human cornea. *Free Radic Biol Med.* 2008;45(8):1047-1055.

75. Tsai YY, Cheng YW, Lee H, et al. Oxidative DNA damage in pterygium. *Mol Vis.* 2005;11: 71-75.

76. Perra MT, Maxia C, Corbu A, et al. Oxidative stress in pterygium: relationship between p53 and 8-hydroxydeoxyguanosine. *Mol Vis.* 2006;12:1136-1142.

77. Kau HC, Tsai CC, Lee CF, et al. Increased oxidative DNA damage, 8-hydroxydeoxy-guanosine, in human pterygium. *Eye.* 2006;20(7):826-831.

78. Lu L, Wang R, Song X. [Pterygium and lipid peroxidation]. *Zhonghua Yan Ke Za Zhi.* 1996;32(3):227-229.

79. Shen A, Ye Y, Wang X, Chen C, Zhang H, Hu J. Raman scattering properties of human pterygium tissue. *J Biomed Opt.* 2005;10(2):024036.

80. Lee DH, Cho HJ, Kim JT, Choi JS, Joo CK. Expression of vascular endothelial growth factor and inducible nitric oxide synthase in pterygia. *Cornea.* 2001;20(7):738-742.

81. Ozdemir G, Inanc F, Kilinc M. Investigation of nitric oxide in pterygium. *Can J Ophthalmol.* 2005;40(6):743-746.

82. Kon K, Fujii S, Kosaka H, Fujiwara T. Nitric oxide synthase inhibition by N(G)-nitro-L-arginine methyl ester retards vascular sprouting in angiogenesis. *Microvasc Res.* 2003;65(1):2-8.

83. Brown DJ, Lin B, Chwa M, Atilano SR, Kim DW, Kenney MC. Elements of the nitric oxide pathway can degrade TIMP-1 and increase gelatinase activity. *Mol Vis.* 2004;10:281-288.

84. Peus D, Vasa RA, Meves A, et al. H_2O_2 is an important mediator of UVB-induced EGF-receptor phosphorylation in cultured keratinocytes. *J Invest Dermatol.* 1998;110(6):966-971.

85. Brenneisen P, Sies H, Scharffetter-Kochanek K. Ultraviolet-B irradiation and matrix metalloproteinases: from induction via signaling to initial events. *Ann NY Acad Sci.* 2002;973:31-43.

86. Di Girolamo N, Wakefield D, Coroneo MT. UVB-mediated induction of cytokines and growth factors in pterygium epithelial cells involves cell surface receptors and intracellular signaling. *Invest Ophthalmol Vis Sci.* 2006;47(6):2430-2437.

87. Di Girolamo N, Coroneo MT, Wakefield D. UVB-elicited induction of MMP-1 expression in human ocular surface epithelial cells is mediated through the ERK1/2 MAPK-dependent pathway. *Invest Ophthalmol Vis Sci.* 2003;44(11):4705-4714.

88. Di Girolamo N, Coroneo M, Wakefield D. Epidermal growth factor receptor signaling is partially responsible for the increased matrix metalloproteinase-1 expression in ocular epithelial cells after UVB radiation. *Am J Pathol.* 2005;167(2):489-503.

89. Wilson SE, Mohan RR, Ambrosio R, Jr., Hong J, Lee J. The corneal wound healing response: cytokine-mediated interaction of the epithelium, stroma, and inflammatory cells. *Prog Retin Eye Res.* 2001;20(5):625-637.

90. Imanishi J, Kamiyama K, Iguchi I, Kita M, Sotozono C, Kinoshita S. Growth factors: importance in wound healing and maintenance of transparency of the cornea. *Prog Retin Eye Res.* 2000;19(1):113-129.

91. Sivak JM, Fini ME. MMPs in the eye: emerging roles for matrix metalloproteinases in ocular physiology. *Prog Retin Eye Res.* 2002;21(1):1-14.

92. Ansel JC, Abraham TA, Zivony AS, Edelhauser HF, Armstrong CA, Song PI. UV induces human corneal epithelial cell NF-κB activation and results in the production of proinflammatory cytokines IL-1, IL-6, IL-8, and TNF-α. *Invest Ophthalmol Vis Sci.* 2001;42(4):S575 abstract 3087.

93. Kennedy M, Kim KH, Harten B, et al. Ultraviolet irradiation induces the production of multiple cytokines by human corneal cells. *Invest Ophthalmol Vis Sci.* 1997;38(12):2483-2491.

94. Di Girolamo N, Kumar RK, Coroneo MT, Wakefield D. UVB-mediated induction of interleukin-6 and -8 in pterygia and cultured human pterygium epithelial cells. *Invest Ophthalmol Vis Sci.* 2002;43(11):3430-3437.

95. Nolan TM, DiGirolamo N, Sachdev NH, Hampartzoumian T, Coroneo MT, Wakefield D. The role of ultraviolet irradiation and heparin-binding epidermal growth factor-like growth factor in the pathogenesis of pterygium. *Am J Pathol.* 2003;162(2):567-574.

96. Blaudschun R, Sunderkotter C, Brenneisen P, et al. Vascular endothelial growth factor causally contributes to the angiogenic response upon ultraviolet B irradiation in vivo. *Br J Dermatol.* 2002;146(4):581-587.

97. Bielenberg DR, Bucana CD, Sanchez R, Donawho CK, Kripke ML, Fidler IJ. Molecular regulation of UVB-induced cutaneous angiogenesis. *J Invest Dermatol.* 1998;111(5):864-872.

98. Ley RD, Miska KB, Kusewitt DF. Photoreactivation of ultraviolet radiation-induced basic fibroblast growth factor (bFGF) and the role of bFGF in corneal lesion formation in Monodelphis domestica. *Environ Mol Mutagen.* 2001;38(2-3):175-179.

99. Baba H, Uchiwa H, Watanabe S. UVB irradiation increases the release of SCF from human epidermal cells. *J Invest Dermatol.* 2005;124(5):1075-1077.

100. Kamel S. The pterygium: its etiology and treatment. *Am J Ophthalmol.* Nov 1954;38(5):682-688.

101. Hill JC, Maske R. Pathogenesis of pterygium. *Eye.* 1989;3(Pt 2):218-226.

102. Omoti AE, Waziri-Erameh JM, Enock ME. Ocular disorders in a petroleum industry in Nigeria. *Eye.* 2008;22(7):925-929.

103. Hilgers JH. Pterygium: its incidence, heredity and etiology. *Am J Ophthalmol.* 1960;50:635-644.

104. Detels R, Dhir SP. Pterygium: a geographical study. *Arch Ophthalmol.* 1967;78(4):485-491.

105. Kubik J. [Our further experiences with pathogenesis of pterigia]. *Ophthalmologica.* 1975;171(3):181-191.

106. Wong WW. A hypothesis on the pathogenesis of pterygiums. *Ann Ophthalmol.* 1978;10(3):303-308.

107. Pinkerton OD, Hokama Y, Shigemura LA. Immunologic basis for the pathogenesis of pterygium. *Am J Ophthalmol.* 1984;98(2):225-228.

108. Liu L, Yang D. Immunological studies on the pathogenesis of pterygium. *Chin Med Sci J.* 1993;8(2):84-88.

109. Liu L. [An immuno-pathological study of pterygium]. *Zhonghua Yan Ke Za Zhi.* 1993;29(3):141-143.

110. Ioachim-Velogianni E, Tsironi E, Agnantis N, Datseris G, Psilas K. HLA-DR antigen expression in pterygium epithelial cells and lymphocyte subpopulations: an immunohistochemistry study. *Ger J Ophthalmol*. 1995;4(2):123-129.

111. Chen YT, Tseng SH, Tsai YY, Huang FC, Tseng SY. Distribution of vimentin-expressing cells in pterygium: an immunocytochemical study of impression cytology specimens. *Cornea*. 2009;28(5):547-552.

112. Tekelioglu Y, Turk A, Avunduk AM, Yulug E. Flow cytometrical analysis of adhesion molecules, T-lymphocyte subpopulations and inflammatory markers in pterygium. *Ophthalmologica*. 2006;220(6): 372-378.

113. Kria L, Ohira A, Amemiya T. Immunohistochemical localization of basic fibroblast growth factor, platelet derived growth factor, transforming growth factor-beta and tumor necrosis factor-alpha in the pterygium. *Acta Histochem*. 1996;98(2):195-201.

114. Wen Z, Liu Z. [The abnormal expression of interleukine-1 family in pterygium]. *Yan Ke Xue Bao*. 2003;19(2):133-136.

115. Kuo CH, Miyazaki D, Yakura K, Araki-Sasaki K, Inoue Y. Role of periostin and interleukin-4 in recurrence of pterygia. *Invest Ophthalmol Vis Sci*. 2010;51(1):139-143.

116. Rundhaug JE, Fischer SM. Cyclo-oxygenase-2 plays a critical role in UV-induced skin carcinogenesis. *Photochem Photobiol*. 2008;84(2):322-329.

117. Chiang CC, Cheng YW, Lin CL, et al. Cyclooxygenase 2 expression in pterygium. *Mol Vis*. 2007;13: 635-638.

118. Karahan N, Baspinar S, Ciris M, Baydar CL, Kapucuoglu N. Cyclooxygenase-2 expression in primary and recurrent pterygium. *Indian J Ophthalmol*. 2008;56(4):279-283.

119. Maxia C, Perra MT, Demurtas P, et al. Relationship between the expression of cyclooxygenase-2 and survivin in primary pterygium. *Mol Vis*. 2009;15:458-463.

120. Ottino P, Bazan HE. Corneal stimulation of MMP-1, -9 and uPA by platelet-activating factor is mediated by cyclo-oxygenase-2 metabolites. *Curr Eye Res*. 2001;23(2):77-85.

121. Eckert RL, Broome AM, Ruse M, Robinson N, Ryan D, Lee K. S100 proteins in the epidermis. *J Invest Dermatol*. 2004;123(1):23-33.

122. Cross SS, Hamdy FC, Deloulme JC, Rehman I. Expression of S100 proteins in normal human tissues and common cancers using tissue microarrays: S100A6, S100A8, S100A9 and S100A11 are all overexpressed in common cancers. *Histopathology*. 2005;46(3):256-269.

123. Riau AK, Wong TT, Beuerman RW, Tong L. Calcium-binding S100 protein expression in pterygium. *Mol Vis*. 2009;15:335-342.

124. Zhou L, Beuerman RW, Ang LP, et al. Elevation of human alpha-defensins and S100 calcium-binding proteins A8 and A9 in tear fluid of patients with pterygium. *Invest Ophthalmol Vis Sci*. 2009;50(5):2077-2086.

125. Marionnet C, Bernerd F, Dumas A, et al. Modulation of gene expression induced in human epidermis by environmental stress in vivo. *J Invest Dermatol*. 2003;121(6):1447-1458.

126. Lee YM, Kim YK, Eun HC, Chung JH. Changes in S100A8 expression in UV-irradiated and aged human skin in vivo. *Arch Dermatol Res*. 2009;301(7):523-529.

127. Lim SY, Raftery MJ, Goyette J, Hsu K, Geczy CL. Oxidative modifications of S100 proteins: functional regulation by redox. *J Leukoc Biol*. 2009;86(3):577-587.

128. Nakagami T, Watanabe I, Murakami A, Okisaka S, Ebihara N. Expression of stem cell factor in pterygium. *Jpn J Ophthalmol*. 2000;44(3):193-197.

129. Lee JK, Song YS, Ha HS, et al. Endothelial progenitor cells in pterygium pathogenesis. *Eye*. 2007;21(9):1186-1193.

130. Butrus SI, Ashraf MF, Laby DM, Rabinowitz AI, Tabbara SO, Hidayat AA. Increased numbers of mast cells in pterygia. *Am J Ophthalmol*. 1995;119(2):236-237.

131. Powers MR, Qu Z, O'Brien B, Wilson DJ, Thompson JE, Rosenbaum JT. Immunolocalization of bFGF in pterygia: association with mast cells. *Cornea*. 1997;16(5):545-549.

132. Ribatti D, Nico B, Maxia C, et al. Neovascularization and mast cells with tryptase activity increase simultaneously in human pterygium. *J Cell Mol Med*. 2007;11(3):585-589.

133. Papadia M, Barabino S, Valente C, Rolando M. Anatomical and immunological changes of the cornea in patients with pterygium. *Curr Eye Res*. 2008;33(5):429-434.

134. Zhivov A, Beck R, Guthoff RF. Corneal and conjunctival findings after mitomycin C application in pterygium surgery: an in-vivo confocal microscopy study. *Acta Ophthalmol*. 2009;87(2):166-172.

135. Labbe A, Gheck L, Iordanidou V, Mehanna C, Brignole-Baudouin F, Baudouin C. An in vivo confocal microscopy and impression cytology evaluation of pterygium activity. *Cornea*. 2010;29(4):392-399.

136. John-Aryankalayil M, Dushku N, Jaworski CJ, et al. Microarray and protein analysis of human pterygium. *Mol Vis*. 2006;12:55-64.

137. Kheirkhah A, Casas V, Sheha H, Raju VK, Tseng SC. Role of conjunctival inflammation in surgical outcome after amniotic membrane transplantation with or without fibrin glue for pterygium. *Cornea*. 2008;27(1):56-63.

138. Aydin A, Karadayi K, Aykan U, Can G, Colakoglu K, Bilge AH. [Effectiveness of topical ciclosporin A treatment after excision of primary pterygium and limbal conjunctival autograft]. *J Fr Ophtalmol*. 2008;31(7):699-704.

139. Wu H, Chen G. [Cyclosporine A and thiotepa in prevention of postoperative recurrence of pterygium]. *Yan Ke Xue Bao*. 1999;15(2):91-92.

140. Awdeh RM, DeStafeno JJ, Blackmon DM, Cummings TJ, Kim T. The presence of T-lymphocyte subpopulations (CD4 and CD8) in pterygia: evaluation of the inflammatory response. *Adv Ther*. 2008;25(5):479-487.

141. Rohrbach IM, Starc S, Knorr M. [Predicting recurrent pterygium based on morphologic and immunohistologic parameters]. *Ophthalmologe*. 1995;92(4):463-468.

142. Garfias Y, Bautista-De Lucio VM, Garcia C, Nava A, Villalvazo L, Jimenez-Martinez MC. Study of the expression of CD30 in pterygia compared to healthy conjunctivas. *Mol Vis*. 2009;15:2068-2073.

143. Kase S, Osaki M, Jin XH, et al. Increased expression of erythropoietin receptor in human pterygial tissues. *Int J Mol Med*. 2007;20(5):699-702.

144. Kria L, Ohira A, Amemiya T. Growth factors in cultured pterygium fibroblasts: immunohistochemical and ELISA analysis. *Graefes Arch Clin Exp Ophthalmol.* 1998;236(9):702-708.

145. Jaworski CJ, Aryankalayil-John M, Campos MM, et al. Expression analysis of human pterygium shows a predominance of conjunctival and limbal markers and genes associated with cell migration. *Mol Vis.* 2009;15:2421-2434.

146. Nolan TM, Di Girolamo N, Coroneo MT, Wakefield D. Proliferative effects of heparin-binding epidermal growth factor-like growth factor on pterygium epithelial cells and fibroblasts. *Invest Ophthalmol Vis Sci.* 2004;45(1):110-113.

147. Liu Z, Xie Y, Zhang M. Overexpression of type I growth factor receptors in pterygium. *Chin Med J (Engl).* 2002;115(3):418-421.

148. Maini R, Collison DJ, Maidment JM, Davies PD, Wormstone IM. Pterygial derived fibroblasts express functionally active histamine and epidermal growth factor receptors. *Exp Eye Res.* 2002;74(2):237-244.

149. Lee SB, Li DQ, Tan DT, Meller DC, Tseng SC. Suppression of TGF-beta signaling in both normal conjunctival fibroblasts and pterygial body fibroblasts by amniotic membrane. *Curr Eye Res.* 2000;20(4):325-334.

150. Hong S, Choi JY, Lee HK, et al. Expression of neurotrophic factors in human primary pterygeal tissue and selective TNF-alpha-induced stimulation of ciliary neurotrophic factor in pterygeal fibroblasts. *Exp Toxicol Pathol.* 2008;60(6):513-520.

151. Ribatti D, Nico B, Perra MT, et al. Correlation between NGF/TrkA and microvascular density in human pterygium. *Int J Exp Pathol.* 2009;90(6):615-620. Epub 2009 Sep 15.

152. Di Girolamo N, Sarris M, Chui J, Cheema H, Coroneo MT, Wakefield D. Localization of the low-affinity nerve growth factor receptor p75 in human limbal epithelial cells. *J Cell Mol Med.* 2008;12(6B):2799-2811.

153. Ren X, Lin YP, Tan DTH, Schultz GS. Elevated expression of TGF-beta and EGF system in pterygia tissues and matched superior conjunctiva (abstract). *Invest Ophthalmol Vis Sci.* 1998:39(suppl):S509.

154. Jin J, Guan M, Sima J, et al. Decreased pigment epithelium-derived factor and increased vascular endothelial growth factor levels in pterygia. *Cornea.* 2003;22(5):473-477.

155. Aspiotis M, Tsanou E, Gorezis S, et al. Angiogenesis in pterygium: study of microvessel density, vascular endothelial growth factor, and thrombospondin-1. *Eye.* 2007;21(8):1095-1101.

156. Marcovich AL, Morad Y, Sandbank J, et al. Angiogenesis in pterygium: morphometric and immunohistochemical study. *Curr Eye Res.* 2002;25(1):17-22.

157. van Setten G, Aspiotis M, Blalock TD, Grotendorst G, Schultz G. Connective tissue growth factor in pterygium: simultaneous presence with vascular endothelial growth factor - possible contributing factor to conjunctival scarring. *Graefes Arch Clin Exp Ophthalmol.* 2003;241(2):135-139.

158. Gebhardt M, Mentlein R, Schaudig U, et al. Differential expression of vascular endothelial growth factor implies the limbal origin of pterygia. *Ophthalmology.* 2005;112(6):1023-1030.

159. Solomon A, Grueterich M, Li DQ, Meller D, Lee SB, Tseng SC. Overexpression of Insulin-like growth factor-binding protein-2 in pterygium body fibroblasts. *Invest Ophthalmol Vis Sci.* 2003;44(2):573-580.

160. Wong YW, Chew J, Yang H, Tan DT, Beuerman R. Expression of insulin-like growth factor binding protein-3 in pterygium tissue. *Br J Ophthalmol.* 2006;90(6):769-772.

161. Abdiu O, Van Setten G. Antiangiogenic activity in tears: presence of pigment-epithelium-derived factor. New insights and preliminary results. *Ophthalmic Res.* 2008;40(1):16-18.

162. Saika S, Yamanaka O, Sumioka T, et al. Fibrotic disorders in the eye: targets of gene therapy. *Prog Retin Eye Res.* 2008;27(2):177-196.

163. Seifert P, Sekundo W. Capillaries in the epithelium of pterygium. *Br J Ophthalmol.* 1998;82(1):77-81.

164. Abramovitch R, Neeman M, Reich R, et al. Intercellular communication between vascular smooth muscle and endothelial cells mediated by heparin-binding epidermal growth factor-like growth factor and vascular endothelial growth factor. *FEBS Lett.* 1998;425(3):441-447.

165. Hernandez GL, Volpert OV, Iniguez MA, et al. Selective inhibition of vascular endothelial growth factor-mediated angiogenesis by cyclosporin A: roles of the nuclear factor of activated T cells and cyclooxygenase 2. *J Exp Med.* 2001;193(5):607-620.

166. Bock F, Onderka J, Dietrich T, et al. Bevacizumab as a potent inhibitor of inflammatory corneal angiogenesis and lymphangiogenesis. *Invest Ophthalmol Vis Sci.* 2007;48(6):2545-2552.

167. Mauro J, Foster CS. Pterygia: pathogenesis and the role of subconjunctival bevacizumab in treatment. *Semin Ophthalmol.* 2009;24(3):130-134.

168. Ansari MW, Rahi AH, Shukla BR. Pseudoelastic nature of pterygium. *Br J Ophthalmol.* 1970;54(7):473-476.

169. Vass Z, Tapaszto I. The histochemical examination of the fibers of pterygium by elastase. *Acta Ophthalmol (Copenh).* 1964;42(4):849-854.

170. Fuchs E. Ueber das pterygium. *Graefes Arch for Ophthalmol.* 1892;38(2):1-89.

171. Duke-Elder S. *Diseases of the Outer Eye Part 1.* Vol 8. London,UK: Henry Kimpton Publishers; 1965:569-585.

172. Di Girolamo N, Wakefield D, Coroneo MT. Differential expression of matrix metalloproteinases and their tissue inhibitors at the advancing pterygium head. *Invest Ophthalmol Vis Sci.* 2000;41(13):4142-4149.

173. Wong TT, Sethi C, Daniels JT, Limb GA, Murphy G, Khaw PT. Matrix metalloproteinases in disease and repair processes in the anterior segment. *Surv Ophthalmol.* 2002;47(3):239-256.

174. Quan T, Qin Z, Xia W, Shao Y, Voorhees JJ, Fisher GJ. Matrix-degrading metalloproteinases in photoaging. *J Investig Dermatol Symp Proc.* 2009;14(1):20-24.

175. Di Girolamo N, McCluskey P, Lloyd A, Coroneo MT, Wakefield D. Expression of MMPs and TIMPs in human pterygia and cultured pterygium epithelial cells. *Invest Ophthalmol Vis Sci.* 2000;41(3):671-679.

176. Solomon A, Li DQ, Lee SB, Tseng SC. Regulation of collagenase, stromelysin, and urokinase-type plasminogen activator in primary pterygium body fibroblasts by inflammatory cytokines. *Invest Ophthalmol Vis Sci.* 2000;41(8):2154-2163.

177. Dushku N, John MK, Schultz GS, Reid TW. Pterygia pathogenesis: corneal invasion by matrix metalloproteinase expressing altered limbal epithelial basal cells. *Arch Ophthalmol.* 2001;119(5):695-706.
178. Di Girolamo N, Coroneo MT, Wakefield D. Active matrilysin (MMP-7) in human pterygia: potential role in angiogenesis. *Invest Ophthalmol Vis Sci.* 2001;42(9):1963-1968.
179. Naib-Majani W, Eltohami I, Wernert N, et al. Distribution of extracellular matrix proteins in pterygia: an immunohistochemical study. *Graefes Arch Clin Exp Ophthalmol.* 2004;242(4):332-338.
180. Li DQ, Lee SB, Gunja-Smith Z, et al. Overexpression of collagenase (MMP-1) and stromelysin (MMP-3) by pterygium head fibroblasts. *Arch Ophthalmol.* 2001;119(1):71-80.
181. Yang SF, Lin CY, Yang PY, Chao SC, Ye YZ, Hu DN. Increased expression of gelatinase (MMP-2 and MMP-9) in pterygia and pterygium fibroblasts with disease progression and activation of protein kinase C. *Invest Ophthalmol Vis Sci.* 2009;50(10):4588-4596.
182. Wang IJ, Hu FR, Chen PJ, Lin CT. Mechanism of abnormal elastin gene expression in the pinguecular part of pterygia. *Am J Pathol.* 2000;157(4):1269-1276.
183. Kaneko M, Takaku I, Katsura N. Glycosaminoglycans in pterygium tissues and normal conjunctiva. *Jpn J Ophthalmol.* 1986;30(2):165-173.
184. Fitzsimmons TD, Molander N, Stenevi U, Fagerholm P, Schenholm M, von Malmborg A. Endogenous hyaluronan in corneal disease. *Invest Ophthalmol Vis Sci.* 1994;35(6):2774-2782.
185. Vlodavsky I, Miao HQ, Medalion B, Danagher P, Ron D. Involvement of heparan sulfate and related molecules in sequestration and growth promoting activity of fibroblast growth factor. *Cancer Metastasis Rev.* 1996;15(2):177-186.
186. Tumova S, Woods A, Couchman JR. Heparan sulfate proteoglycans on the cell surface: versatile coordinators of cellular functions. *Int J Biochem Cell Biol.* 2000;32(3):269-288.
187. Dua HS, Azuara-Blanco A. Limbal stem cells of the corneal epithelium. *Surv Ophthalmol.* 2000;44(5):415-425.
188. Lavker RM, Tseng SC, Sun TT. Corneal epithelial stem cells at the limbus: looking at some old problems from a new angle. *Exp Eye Res.* 2004;78(3):433-446.
189. Dushku N, Reid TW. Immunohistochemical evidence that human pterygia originate from an invasion of vimentin-expressing altered limbal epithelial basal cells. *Curr Eye Res.* 1994;13(7):473-481.
190. Kato N, Shimmura S, Kawakita T, et al. Beta-catenin activation and epithelial-mesenchymal transition in the pathogenesis of pterygium. *Invest Ophthalmol Vis Sci.* 2007;48(4):1511-1517.
191. Park TK, Jin KH. Telomerase activity in pterygeal and normal conjunctival epithelium. *Korean J Ophthalmol.* 2000;14(2):85-89.
192. Shimmura S, Ishioka M, Hanada K, Shimazaki J, Tsubota K. Telomerase activity and p53 expression in pterygia. *Invest Ophthalmol Vis Sci.* 2000;41(6):1364-1369.
193. Sakoonwatanyoo P, Tan DT, Smith DR. Expression of p63 in pterygium and normal conjunctiva. *Cornea.* 2004;23(1):67-70.
194. Pellegrini G, Dellambra E, Golisano O, et al. p63 identifies keratinocyte stem cells. *Proc Natl Acad Sci USA.* 2001;98(6):3156-3161.
195. Atkinson SD, Moore JE, Shah S, et al. P63 expression in conjunctival proliferative diseases: pterygium and laryngo-onycho-cutaneous (LOC) syndrome. *Curr Eye Res.* 2008;33(7):551-558.
196. Wang IJ, Lai WT, Liou SW, et al. Impression cytology of pterygium. *J Ocul Pharmacol Ther.* 2000;16(6):519-528.
197. Chan CM, Liu YP, Tan DT. Ocular surface changes in pterygium. *Cornea.* 2002;21(1):38-42.
198. Ma DH, Chen JK, Zhang F, Lin KY, Yao JY, Yu JS. Regulation of corneal angiogenesis in limbal stem cell deficiency. *Prog Retin Eye Res.* 2006;25(6):563-590.
199. Vojnikovic B, Njiric S, Zamolo G, Toth I, Apanjol J, Coklo M. Histopathology of the pterygium in population on Croatian Island Rab. *Coll Antropol.* 2007;31(suppl 1):39-41.
200. Dekaris I, Gabric N, Karaman Z, Mravicic I, Kastelan S, Spoljaric N. Pterygium treatment with limbal-conjunctival autograft transplantation. *Coll Antropol.* 2001;25(suppl):7-12.
201. Tan D. Conjunctival grafting for ocular surface disease. *Curr Opin Ophthalmol.* 1999;10(4): 277-281.
202. Kase S, Osaki M, Sato I, et al. Immunolocalisation of E-cadherin and beta-catenin in human pterygium. *Br J Ophthalmol.* 2007;91(9):1209-1212.
203. Zavadil J, Bottinger EP. TGF-beta and epithelial-to-mesenchymal transitions. *Oncogene.* 2005;24(37):5764-5774.
204. Strutz F, Zeisberg M, Ziyadeh FN, et al. Role of basic fibroblast growth factor-2 in epithelial-mesenchymal transformation. *Kidney Int.* 2002;61(5):1714-1728.
205. Hudson LG, Choi C, Newkirk KM, et al. Ultraviolet radiation stimulates expression of Snail family transcription factors in keratinocytes. *Mol Carcinog.* 2007;46(4):257-268.
206. Touhami A, Di Pascuale MA, Kawatika T, et al. Characterisation of myofibroblasts in fibrovascular tissues of primary and recurrent pterygia. *Br J Ophthalmol.* 2005;89(3):269-274.
207. Ye J, Song YS, Kang SH, Yao K, Kim JC. Involvement of bone marrow-derived stem and progenitor cells in the pathogenesis of pterygium. *Eye.* 2004;18(8):839-843.
208. Song YS, Ryu YH, Choi SR, Kim JC. The involvement of adult stem cells originated from bone marrow in the pathogenesis of pterygia. *Yonsei Med J.* 2005;46(5):687-692.
209. Yamagami S, Ebihara N, Usui T, Yokoo S, Amano S. Bone marrow-derived cells in normal human corneal stroma. *Arch Ophthalmol.* 2006;124(1):62-69.
210. Ishii G, Sangai T, Sugiyama K, et al. In vivo characterization of bone marrow-derived fibroblasts recruited into fibrotic lesions. *Stem Cells.* 2005;23(5):699-706.
211. Takahashi T, Kalka C, Masuda H, et al. Ischemia- and cytokine-induced mobilization of bone marrow-derived endothelial progenitor cells for neovascularization. *Nat Med.* 1999;5(4):434-438.
212. Sevel D, Sealy R. Pterygia and carcinoma of the conjunctiva. *Trans Ophthalmol Soc UK.* 1969;88: 567-578.

213. Hirst LW, Axelsen RA, Schwab I. Pterygium and associated ocular surface squamous neoplasia. *Arch Ophthalmol.* 2009;127(1):31-32.
214. Perra MT, Colombari R, Maxia C, et al. Finding of conjunctival melanocytic pigmented lesions within pterygium. *Histopathology.* 2006;48(4):387-393.
215. Tan DT, Tang WY, Liu YP, Goh HS, Smith DR. Apoptosis and apoptosis related gene expression in normal conjunctiva and pterygium. *Br J Ophthalmol.* 2000;84(2):212-216.
216. Tsironi S, Ioachim E, Machera M, Aspiotis M, Agnanti N, Psilas K. Presence and possible significance of immunohistochemically demonstrable metallothionein expression in pterygium versus pinguecula and normal conjunctiva. *Eye.* 2001;15(Pt 1):89-96.
217. Ueda Y, Kanazawa S, Kitaoka T, et al. Immunohistochemical study of p53, p21 and PCNA in pterygium. *Acta Histochem.* 2001;103(2):159-165.
218. Kase S, Takahashi S, Sato I, Nakanishi K, Yoshida K, Ohno S. Expression of p27(KIP1) and cyclin D1, and cell proliferation in human pterygium. *Br J Ophthalmol.* 2007;91(7):958-961.
219. Tan DT, Liu YP, Sun L. Flow cytometry measurements of DNA content in primary and recurrent pterygia. *Invest Ophthalmol Vis Sci.* 2000;41(7):1684-1686.
220. Chen JK, Tsai RJ, Lin SS. Fibroblasts isolated from human pterygia exhibit transformed cell characteristics. *In Vitro Cell Dev Biol Anim.* 1994;30A(4):243-248.
221. Peiretti E, Dessi S, Mulas MF, Abete C, Galantuomo MS, Fossarello M. Fibroblasts isolated from human pterygia exhibit altered lipid metabolism characteristics. *Exp Eye Res.* 2006;83(3):536-542.
222. Lee KW, Cohen P. Nuclear effects: unexpected intracellular actions of insulin-like growth factor binding protein-3. *J Endocrinol.* 2002;175(1):33-40.
223. Booth F. Heredity in one hundred patients admitted for excision of pterygia. *Aust NZ J Ophthalmol.* 1985;13(1):59-61.
224. Islam SI, Wagoner MD. Pterygium in young members of one family. *Cornea.* 2001;20(7):708-710.
225. Carmichael TR. Genetic factors in pterygium in South Africans. *S Afr Med J.* 2001;91(4):322.
226. Bloom AH, Perry HD, Donnenfeld ED, Pinchoff BS, Solomon R. Childhood onset of pterygia in twins. *Eye Contact Lens.* 2005;31(6):279-280.
227. Zhang JD. An investigation of aetiology and heredity of pterygium. Report of 11 cases in a family. *Acta Ophthalmol (Copenh).* 1987;65(4):413-416.
228. Hecht F, Shoptaugh MG. Winglets of the eye: dominant transmission of early adult pterygium of the conjunctiva. *J Med Genet.* 1990;27(6):392-394.
229. Goyal JL, Rao VA, Srinivasan R, Agrawal K. Oculocutaneous manifestations in xeroderma pigmentosa. *Br J Ophthalmol.* 1994;78(4):295-297.
230. Kau HC, Tsai CC, Hsu WM, Liu JH, Wei YH. Genetic polymorphism of hOGG1 and risk of pterygium in Chinese. *Eye.* 2004;18(6):635-639.
231. Tsai YY, Lee H, Tseng SH, et al. Null type of glutathione S-transferase M1 polymorphism is associated with early onset pterygium. *Mol Vis.* 2004;10:458-461.
232. Tsai YY, Bau DT, Chiang CC, Cheng YW, Tseng SH, Tsai FJ. Pterygium and genetic polymorphism of DNA double strand break repair gene Ku70. *Mol Vis.* 2007;13:1436-1440.
233. Tsai YY, Cheng YW, Lee H, Tseng SH, Tsai CH, Tsai FJ. No association of p53 codon 72 and p21 codon 31 polymorphisms in Taiwan Chinese patients with pterygium. *Br J Ophthalmol.* 2004;88(7):975-976.
234. Tsai YY, Chang KC, Lee H, et al. Effect of p53 codon 72 polymorphism on p53 protein expression in pterygium. *Clin Experiment Ophthalmol.* 2005;33(1):60-62.
235. Rodrigues FW, Arruda JT, Silva RE, Moura KK. TP53 gene expression, codon 72 polymorphism and human papillomavirus DNA associated with pterygium. *Genet Mol Res.* 2008;7(4):1251-1258.
236. Tsai YY, Lee H, Tseng SH, et al. Evaluation of TNF-alpha and IL-1beta polymorphisms in Taiwan Chinese patients with pterygium. *Eye.* 2005;19(5):571-574.
237. Tsai YY, Chiang CC, Bau DT, et al. Vascular endothelial growth factor gene 460 polymorphism is associated with pterygium formation in female patients. *Cornea.* 2008;27(4):476-479.
238. Bau DT, Chiang CC, Tsai YY, et al. Evaluation of transforming growth factor and vascular endothelial growth factor polymorphisms in Taiwan Chinese patients with pterygium. *Eur J Ophthalmol.* 2008;18(1):21-26.
239. Spandidos DA, Sourvinos G, Kiaris H, Tsamparlakis J. Microsatellite instability and loss of heterozygosity in human pterygia. *Br J Ophthalmol.* 1997;81(6):493-496.
240. Detorakis ET, Zafiropoulos A, Arvanitis DA, Spandidos DA. Detection of point mutations at codon 12 of KI-ras in ophthalmic pterygia. *Eye.* 2005;19(2):210-214.
241. Tsai YY, Cheng YW, Lee H, Tsai FJ, Tseng SH, Chang KC. P53 gene mutation spectrum and the relationship between gene mutation and protein levels in pterygium. *Mol Vis.* 2005;11:50-55.
242. Tsai YY, Chang CC, Chiang CC, et al. HPV infection and p53 inactivation in pterygium. *Mol Vis.* 2009;15:1092-1097.
243. Reisman D, McFadden JW, Lu G. Loss of heterozygosity and p53 expression in Pterygium. *Cancer Lett.* 2004;206(1):77-83.
244. Chen PL, Cheng YW, Chiang CC, Tseng SH, Chau PS, Tsai YY. Hypermethylation of the p16 gene promoter in pterygia and its association with the expression of DNA methyltransferase 3b. *Mol Vis.* 2006;12:1411-1416.
245. Lakin ND, Jackson SP. Regulation of p53 in response to DNA damage. *Oncogene.* 1999;18(53):7644-7655.
246. Drouin R, Therrien JP. UVB-induced cyclobutane pyrimidine dimer frequency correlates with skin cancer mutational hotspots in p53. *Photochem Photobiol.* 1997;66(5):719-726.
247. Dushku N, Reid TW. P53 expression in altered limbal basal cells of pingueculae, pterygia, and limbal tumors. *Curr Eye Res.* 1997;16(12):1179-1192.

248. Tan DT, Lim AS, Goh HS, Smith DR. Abnormal expression of the p53 tumor suppressor gene in the conjunctiva of patients with pterygium. *Am J Ophthalmol.* 1997;123(3):404-405.

249. Chowers I, Pe'er J, Zamir E, Livni N, Ilsar M, Frucht-Pery J. Proliferative activity and p53 expression in primary and recurrent pterygia. *Ophthalmology.* 2001;108(5):985-988.

250. Weinstein O, Rosenthal G, Zirkin H, Monos T, Lifshitz T, Argov S. Overexpression of p53 tumor suppressor gene in pterygia. *Eye.* 2002;16(5):619-621.

251. Pelit A, Bal N, Akova YA, Demirhan B. p53 expression in pterygium in two climatic regions in Turkey. *Indian J Ophthalmol.* 2009;57(3):203-206.

252. Onur C, Orhan D, Orhan M, Dizbay Sak S, Tulunay O, Irkec M. Expression of p53 protein in pterygium. *Eur J Ophthalmol.* 1998;8(3):157-161.

253. Schneider BG, John-Aryankalayil M, Rowsey JJ, Dushku N, Reid TW. Accumulation of p53 protein in pterygia is not accompanied by TP53 gene mutation. *Exp Eye Res.* 2006;82(1):91-98.

254. Detorakis ET, Drakonaki EE, Spandidos DA. Molecular genetic alterations and viral presence in ophthalmic pterygium. *Int J Mol Med.* 2000;6(1):35-41.

255. Piras F, Moore PS, Ugalde J, Perra MT, Scarpa A, Sirigu P. Detection of human papillomavirus DNA in pterygia from different geographical regions. *Br J Ophthalmol.* 2003;87(7):864-866.

256. Chen KH, Hsu WM, Cheng CC, Li YS. Lack of human papillomavirus in pterygium of Chinese patients from Taiwan. *Br J Ophthalmol.* 2003;87(8):1046-1048.

257. Dushku N, Hatcher SL, Albert DM, Reid TW. p53 expression and relation to human papillomavirus infection in pingueculae, pterygia, and limbal tumors. *Arch Ophthalmol.* 1999;117(12):1593-1599.

258. Schellini SA, Hoyama E, Shiratori CA, Sakamoto RH, Candeias JM. Lack of papillomavirus (HPV) in pterygia of a Brazilian sample. *Arq Bras Oftalmol.* 2006;69(4):519-521.

259. Guthoff R, Marx A, Stroebel P. No evidence for a pathogenic role of human papillomavirus infection in ocular surface squamous neoplasia in Germany. *Curr Eye Res.* 2009;34(8):666-671.

260. Detorakis ET, Sourvinos G, Spandidos DA. Detection of herpes simplex virus and human papilloma virus in ophthalmic pterygium. *Cornea.* 2001;20(2):164-167.

261. Chen YF, Hsiao CH, Ngan KW, et al. Herpes simplex virus and pterygium in Taiwan. *Cornea.* 2008;27(3):311-313.

262. Chui J, Di Girolamo N, Coroneo MT, Wakefield D. The role of substance P in the pathogenesis of pterygia. *Invest Ophthalmol Vis Sci.* 2007;48(10):4482-4489.

263. Thoft RA, Friend J. The X, Y, Z hypothesis of corneal epithelial maintenance. *Invest Ophthalmol Vis Sci.* 1983;24(10):1442-1443.

264. Muller LJ, Marfurt CF, Kruse F, Tervo TM. Corneal nerves: structure, contents and function. *Exp Eye Res.* 2003;76(5):521-542.

265. Benrath J, Zimmermann M, Gillardon F. Substance P and nitric oxide mediate would healing of ultraviolet photo-damaged rat skin: evidence for an effect of nitric oxide on keratinocyte proliferation. *Neurosci Lett.* 1995;200(1):17-20.

266. Ansel JC, Armstrong CA, Song I, et al. Interactions of the skin and nervous system. *J Investig Dermatol Symp Proc.* 1997;2(1):23-26.

267. Luger TA, Lotti T. Neuropeptides: role in inflammatory skin diseases. *J Eur Acad Dermatol Venereol.* 1998;10(3):207-211.

268. Legat FJ, Griesbacher T, Schicho R, et al. Repeated subinflammatory ultraviolet B irradiation increases substance P and calcitonin gene-related peptide content and augments mustard oil-induced neurogenic inflammation in the skin of rats. *Neurosci Lett.* 2002;329(3):309-313.

269. van der Zypen F, van der Zypen E, Daicker B. [Ultrastructural studies on the pterygium. II. Connective tissue, vessels and nerves of the conjunctival part (author's transl)]. *Albrecht Von Graefes Arch Klin Exp Ophthalmol.* 1975;193(3):177-187.

270. Karukonda SR, Thompson HW, Beuerman RW, et al. Cell cycle kinetics in pterygium at three latitudes. *Br J Ophthalmol.* 1995;79(4):313-317.

271. Gallagher MJ, Giannoudis A, Herrington CS, Hiscott P. Human papillomavirus in pterygium. *Br J Ophthalmol.* 2001;85(7):782-784.

272. Sjo NC, von Buchwald C, Prause JU, Norrild B, Vinding T, Heegaard S. Human papillomavirus and pterygium. Is the virus a risk factor? *Br J Ophthalmol.* 2007;91(8):1016-1018.

273. Takamura Y, Kubo E, Tsuzuki S, Akagi Y. Detection of human papillomavirus in pterygium and conjunctival papilloma by hybrid capture II and PCR assays. *Eye.* 2008;22(11):1442-1445.

274. Otlu B, Emre S, Turkcuoglu P, Doganay S, Durmaz R. Investigation of human papillomavirus and Epstein-Barr virus DNAs in pterygium tissue. *Eur J Ophthalmol.* 2009;19(2):175-179.

275. Piecyk-Sidor M, Polz-Dacewicz M, Zagorski Z, Zarnowski T. Occurrence of human papillomavirus in pterygia. *Acta Ophthalmol.* 2009;87(8):890-895.

276. Hsiao CH, Lee BH, Ngan KW, et al. Presence of human papillomavirus in pterygium in Taiwan. *Cornea.* 2010;29(2):123-127.

277. Kobayashi A, Sugiyama K. In vivo corneal confocal microscopic findings of palisades of Vogt and its underlying limbal stroma. *Cornea.* 2005;24(4):435-437.

278. Ueda S, del Cerro M, LoCascio JA, Aquavella JV. Peptidergic and catecholaminergic fibers in the human corneal epithelium. An immunohistochemical and electron microscopic study. *Acta Ophthalmol Suppl.* 1989;192:80-90.

279. Tan DT, Chee SP, Dear KB, Lim AS. Effect of pterygium morphology on pterygium recurrence in a controlled trial comparing conjunctival autografting with bare sclera excision. *Arch Ophthalmol.* 1997;115(10):1235-1240.

280. Kandavel R, Kang JJ, Memarzadeh F, Chuck RS. Comparison of pterygium recurrence rates in Hispanic and white patients after primary excision and conjunctival autograft. *Cornea.* 2010;29(2):141-145.

281. Detorakis ET, Sourvinos G, Tsamparlakis J, Spandidos DA. Evaluation of loss of heterozygosity and microsatellite instability in human pterygium: clinical correlations. *Br J Ophthalmol.* 1998;82(11):1324-1328.
282. Viveiros MM, Schellini SA, Rogato S, Rainho C, Padovani CR. [Fibroblasts from primary and recurrent pterygia and Tenon's capsule in cell culture]. *Arq Bras Oftalmol.* 2006;69(1):57-62.
283. Ramalho FS, Maestri C, Ramalho LN, Ribeiro-Silva A, Romao E. Expression of p63 and p16 in primary and recurrent pterygia. *Graefes Arch Clin Exp Ophthalmol.* 2006;244(10):1310-1314.
284. Kuo CH, Miyazaki D, Nawata N, et al. Prognosis-determinant candidate genes identified by whole genome scanning in eyes with pterygia. *Invest Ophthalmol Vis Sci.* 2007;48(8):3566-3575.
285. Tong L, Chew J, Yang H, Ang LP, Tan DT, Beuerman RW. Distinct gene subsets in pterygia formation and recurrence: dissecting complex biological phenomenon using genome wide expression data. *BMC Med Genomics.* 2009;2:14.

2

Historical Approaches to Pterygium Surgery, Including Bare Sclera and Adjunctive Beta Radiation Techniques

R. Duncan Johnson, MD; Vicky C. Pai, MD; and Richard H. Hoft, MD

A pterygium is a relatively common, and yet also enigmatic, condition that has been studied by practitioners of medicine and surgery for more than 2000 years. This chapter will briefly review some of the earliest attempts to surgically treat this disorder. Other more recent techniques, developed and used during the 19th and early 20th centuries, will also be reviewed. In some instances, the earliest reports of techniques that are accepted and widely used today (and discussed in more detail in other chapters of this book) will be presented in this chapter.

Antiquity and the Middle Ages

Pterygium, a Latin term derived from the Greek word meaning "small wing," is mentioned frequently and with extraordinary accuracy in ancient Greek, Arabian, Indian, Chinese, and Medieval medical manuscripts. However, the management of pterygium in the ancient world was extremely problematic. Those who described its medical and surgical management, including Hippocrates, Celsus, Pallus, Sushruta, and Aetius, among others, discussed the innate difficulties, with an abundance of complications and its tendency to recur.

Celsus (c. 25 AD) was among the first to record a surgical approach.[1] He describes a procedure in which needle and thread are passed underneath the pterygium (which he called *unguis*—translated as "the claw"). The thread is then elevated and, using a sawing action, the full extent of the pterygium is elevated from the cornea to the canthus. All of the elevated tissue would then be excised with a knife. This surgery was, however, fraught with complications that often caused further pain and blindness. Later, Georg Bartisch (1535-1607 AD) advised that pterygium surgery should be "only rarely done because of the danger to the eye."[2] Ambroise Paré, another 16th century physician, noted that "a pterygium is an illness that always recurs, even when you have done everything in your power to cure it."[3] Indeed, this sentiment still has an element of truth today.

Hovanesian JA. *Pterygium: Techniques and Technologies for Surgical Success (pp 27-36).*
© 2012 Taylor & Francis Group

Nineteenth and Early Twentieth Century

The plethora of surgical treatments used for pterygium from 1800 through the 1930s attest to the fact that the treatment methods during this time were neither very effective nor successful. Surgeons during this period tried many variations of techniques, including excision, incision, cauterization, transplantation, redirection, surgical division or splitting, inversion, irradiation, coagulation, rotation, and chemical treatment. Each of these techniques was also combined with various methods of conjunctival closure.

Excision With Simple Conjunctival Closure

The most common technique of excision with simple conjunctival closure was first described by Arlt in the mid-1800s.[4] In this technique, the pterygium was shaved off the cornea, and then the affected conjunctiva was removed from the limbus to the caruncle. The bulbar conjunctival defect was then closed with vertically-placed interrupted sutures (Figure 2-1). Fuchs stated that care must especially be taken in the closure of the conjunctiva near the limbus or the conjunctiva will grow over the raw surface of the cornea and cause a recurrence of the pterygium. Hirst, in a review of relevant literature, stated that the recurrence rate after simple conjunctival closure was between 45% and 70% in well-designed studies.[5] The simplicity of this procedure results in fast and effective short-term results with very few operative complications. However, the high frequency of recurrence was undesirable and unsatisfactory.

Transplantation/Redirection

In an attempt to lessen the frequency of recurrence, various other methods were tried at the beginning of the 20th century. Redirection, or transplantation of the pterygium head away from the cornea, became the most popular and widely used method during the first half of the 20th century. This technique was first described by Desmarres in the middle of the 19th century,[3] but a variation of the technique described by McReynolds in 1902 became most popular.[6] In this operation, the head of the pterygium was removed from the cornea and then redirected inferiorly, underneath the inferonasal bulbar conjunctiva, and secured into the lower fornix with sutures. Multiple variations of McReynolds' technique were described, including redirection of the pterygium head superiorly[7]; splitting the head, then redirecting the superior portion into the superior fornix and the inferior portion into the inferior fornix[8]; and some surgeons even advocated folding the pterygium back to direct the head toward the caruncle.[9]

The technique of pterygium redirection had the advantage of not removing any conjunctiva as well as being a quick and relatively simple procedure. However, the results were often unsatisfactory because the redirected pterygium head would frequently cause a large, unsightly, and cosmetically unacceptable subconjunctival mass.

Several authors who promoted redirection of the pterygium had postulated that the head of the pterygium was the source of growth. Thus, if the advancing pterygium head was detached and redirected elsewhere, these authors expected the pterygium would grow away from the visual axis. This assumption, however, proved to be incorrect. Recurrent growth of pterygium tissue onto the peripheral cornea was reported to be in the range of 30% to 50%.[10] Most surgeons, therefore, eventually abandoned this technique.

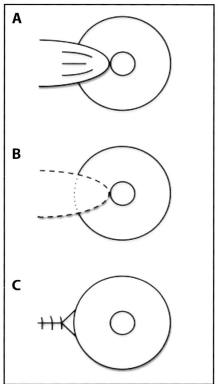

Figure 2-1. Simple closure technique. (A) Large nasal pterygium. (B) Pterygium excised from cornea and adjacent nasal anterior sclera. (C) Bulbar conjunctival defect created by pterygium excision is then closed by pulling superior and inferior conjunctiva together and securing the conjunctiva in its new position with 3 vertical sutures. (Illustration created by Vicky C. Pai, MD and Mr. Chuck Feldman.)

Mid-Twentieth Century and Later

Bare Sclera Technique

A significant change in the surgical management of pterygia occurred in the late 1940s as the failure of the redirection technique became obvious. In 1948, D'Ombrain described a new procedure that eventually evolved into what is now called the *bare sclera technique*.[11] This method consisted of complete excision of the pterygium head as well as removal of at least some of the adjacent abnormal nasal bulbar conjunctiva. Tenon's tissue underlying the area from which abnormal nasal bulbar conjunctiva had been removed was then also excised, thus "baring the sclera." The surrounding normal bulbar conjunctiva was then sutured directly to the sclera, leaving an area of bare sclera at least several millimeters in width adjacent to the limbus (Figure 2-2). This technique was developed to allow the corneal epithelium to heal before the conjunctival epithelium was able to heal over the area of bare sclera and reach the limbus. Other surgeons subsequently made many adjustments to this technique.[12,13]

The bare sclera technique was also a relatively quick and simple procedure. Complications associated with this technique (other than recurrence) were infrequent. However, the rate of pterygium recurrence was still unacceptably high.[14,15] The bare sclera technique is still used today by some surgeons, although usually in combination with adjunctive radiation or antimetabolite treatment.

Figure 2-2. Bare sclera technique. (A) Large nasal pterygium. (B) Pterygium excised from cornea, and pterygium and underlying Tenon's tissue excised from adjacent nasal anterior sclera. (C) The conjunctiva surrounding the area of pterygium and Tenon's tissue excision is secured with sutures, resulting in an area of bare sclera adjacent to the nasal limbus. (Illustration created by Vicky C. Pai, MD and Mr. Chuck Feldman.)

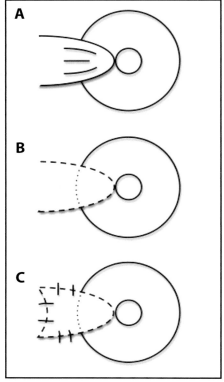

Bare Sclera Technique Combined With Adjunctive Radiation or Chemotherapy

Beta irradiation is a form of ionizing radiation that emits high-energy, high-speed electrons that are rapidly attenuated by biological tissues, depending upon the type of radioactive nuclei used. Beta irradiation was first introduced as a useful tool in ophthalmology by Illiff in 1948, but at that time, its utility was limited by the need to use naturally occurring radon.[16] Three years later, in 1951, the first clinical use of a Strontium-90 (Sr) applicator in ophthalmology was described.[17] Rosenthal subsequently demonstrated the use of a Sr-90 source for treatment of pterygia in 1953.[18] The use of beta radiation for pterygium treatment became popular in the 1970s, especially in Australia and the United States.[19]

The treatment of pterygia with beta irradiation was usually performed after excision of the pterygium using a variation of the bare sclera technique. Pterygium excision was followed by placement of a beta ray plaque, which was most commonly a Sr-90 source, either immediately or within a few days after surgery (Figure 2-3). The total radiation dose varied from 1000 to 7000 centigray (cGy). The total dose was given in a single application, or in fractions given over a period of several weeks.[20] One study analyzing single versus fractionated treatment found a higher therapeutic ratio in patients receiving fractionated treatment.[21] The recurrence rates for pterygium excision with beta irradiation ranged from 0.5% to 52%.[22] A large retrospective study of 825 patients in Florida with excision of primary or recurrent pterygia followed by 6000 cGy of Sr-90 reported a recurrence rate of 1.7% after a mean follow-up period of 8 years.[23] A randomized, double-blind study from the Netherlands of 86 primary

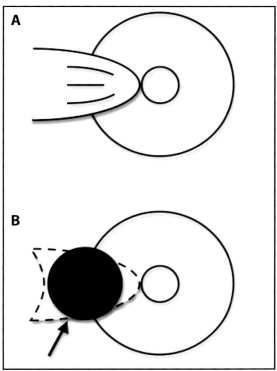

Figure 2-3. Bare sclera technique followed by beta irradiation. (A) Large nasal pterygium. (B) After excision of the pterygium using the bare sclera technique, a Sr-90 plaque (represented by the solid black circle) is applied to the area of excision for an appropriate length of time to deliver a specified dose of beta irradiation. (Illustration created by Vicky C. Pai, MD and Mr. Chuck Feldman.)

pterygia that compared bare sclera excision followed by 2500 cGy of Sr-90 beta irradiation to bare sclera excision and sham irradiation found recurrence rates of 11% and 76%, respectively, with a mean follow-up interval of 21 months (p<0.001).[24]

The complications of beta irradiation treatment after pterygium excision include conjunctivitis, punctate keratitis, cataract, scleromalacia, infectious scleritis, and (rarely) endophthalmitis.[19] Several studies have reported the development of *Streptococcus pneumoniae*-necrotizing scleritis as early as 2 weeks or as late as 13 years after beta radiation treatment.[25,26] A large retrospective study from Australia using an average dose of 2200 cGy (with a follow-up interval ranging between 3 months and 10 years) found that 13% of the study subjects developed some degree of scleromalacia. Four and a half percent of the patients in this same study developed severe scleral thinning, which was defined as at least 50% loss of normal sclera thickness.[27] Some studies have shown a positive correlation between the frequency and severity of complications and the total dose of radiation administered. Severe complications, however, can occasionally occur with relatively low doses of beta irradiation.[19,28] Although the risk of severe and even catastrophic complications from beta radiation treatment is relatively low, many surgeons decided that the risks outweighed the benefits when pterygium surgery was performed primarily for cosmetic reasons.

Triethylene thiophosphoramide, or thiotepa, a radiomimetic alkylating agent, was also used as an adjunctive treatment for pterygium. The use of thiotepa appears to have started at approximately the same time as beta irradiation therapy, although the use of thiotepa is less well documented.

Postoperative administration as an eye drop after bare sclera excision was most common. The usual dose was a dilution of 1:2000 given 4 to 6 times daily for 4 to 6 weeks.[22] Relatively few studies are available concerning the rate of pterygium recurrence after treatment with thiotepa. One study reported a recurrence rate of 3%, while the results of another study indicated that the rate of recurrence was 28%.[29,30] Complications from thiotepa treatment appeared to have been very infrequent, but there was one report of *Pseudomonas aeruginosa* corneoscleritis.[26] The use of this chemotherapeutic agent has diminished over time due to the advent of treatments discussed elsewhere in this book.

Pterygium Excision Combined With Sliding or Pedicle Flaps

Many surgeons have used techniques other than simple conjunctival closure to mobilize, and rearrange, the surrounding normal conjunctiva in order to partially or completely close a bulbar conjunctival defect created by pterygium excision. These techniques have many variations and names. Some of the more common terms, for example, are sliding conjunctival flaps, pedicle flaps or grafts, conjunctival Z-plasty, conjunctivoplasty, and conjunctival relaxing incisions. The review article by Hirst has illustrations of a simple sliding conjunctival flap technique and conjunctival Z-plasty.[22] Figure 2-4 illustrates a more complex variation of a sliding flap technique presently used by one of the authors (Dr. Richard H. Hoft) for conjunctival closure after excision of relatively small, and primary (not recurrent), pterygia.

Sliding flap techniques are also useful for partial closure of large conjunctival defects created by excision of large pterygia. The defect can be made smaller by mobilization and repositioning of surrounding normal conjunctiva. If desired, a free conjunctival autograft, or an amniotic membrane graft, can then be placed in the remaining bulbar conjunctival defect. This method is helpful when the bulbar conjunctival defect created by pterygium excision is very large, and there is an insufficient amount of free conjunctival (or amniotic membrane) graft tissue available to completely cover and close the defect created by surgical excision of the pterygium.

Graft Tissue for Pterygium Surgery

The concept and actual use of graft tissue during pterygium surgery is not new. In 1876, Klein described the use of a mucous membrane graft to cover the defect created by pterygium surgery.[31] In 1926, Elschnig used conjunctival graft tissue from the eye undergoing pterygium excision,[32] while Gomez-Marquez described harvesting conjunctiva from the superior bulbar region of the fellow eye in 1931.[33] In 1977, after Thoft published his landmark article describing the use of conjunctival autografts for various corneal and conjunctival surface disorders, there was renewed interest in the use of conjunctiva autografts for pterygium surgery.[34] The technique of Kenyon and associates, published in 1985, was the basis for the most common technique for pterygium surgery combined with conjunctival autograft that is still widely used today.[35]

Grafts used for pterygium surgery, however, were not limited to only conjunctiva and mucous membrane tissue. Split-thickness skin graft tissue was used by Hotz in 1892[36] and Gifford in 1909.[37] These surgeons reported reasonably good results with their techniques; it is unclear why their methods were never more widely used.

The use of lamellar corneal graft tissue in pterygium surgery was first described by Magitot in 1916.[38] Various other authors have more recently published reports concerning this technique.[39-41] This method has never been widely used, most probably because it is more complex and time consuming, and requires more expensive graft tissue than other available methods. One technique for performing a lamellar corneoscleral graft during pterygium surgery is illustrated in Figure 2-5.

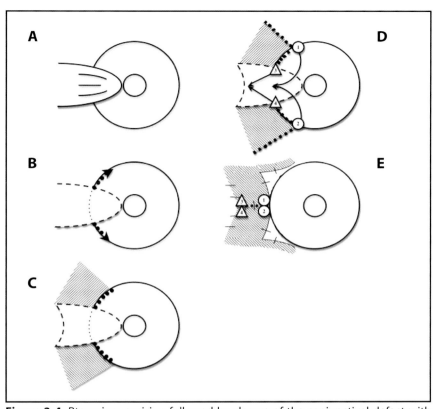

Figure 2-4. Pterygium excision followed by closure of the conjunctival defect with sliding or pedicle flaps. (A) Large nasal pterygium. (B) After pterygium excision, normal conjunctiva is separated from the limbus for 4 to 8 mm superior and inferior to the area of pterygium excision. (These superior and inferior limbal peritomies are represented with arrows followed by 3 large black dots.) (C) The shaded areas of conjunctiva superior and inferior to the area of pterygium excision are undermined with blunt and sharp dissection to separate the conjunctiva from underlying Tenon's and sclera tissue. (D) At the superior termination of the superior peritomy and the inferior termination of the inferior peritomy, incisions are made in the conjunctiva, in a direction radial to the limbus, to separate the areas of undermined conjunctiva from adjacent conjunctival tissue. (The 2 radial incisions are represented by a row of small squares extending radially, or peripherally, from the superior and inferior extent, respectively, of the superior and inferior areas of undermined conjunctiva.) The superior conjunctival flap is then rotated inferiorly and the inferior conjunctival flap is rotated superiorly in a manner that first brings points 3 and 4 together. Points 1 and 2 are then brought together at a location that is more near to the limbus than points 3 and 4. (E) The 2 conjunctival flaps are secured in their new positions with interrupted sutures and/or tissue adhesive. (Illustration created by Vicky C. Pai, MD and Mr. Chuck Feldman.)

Panzardi first described the use of amniotic membrane grafts for pterygium surgery in 1947.[42] Other chapters in this text describe the most recent methods for using amniotic membrane grafts in pterygium surgery and the important contributions of recent investigators and innovators to these contemporary methods.

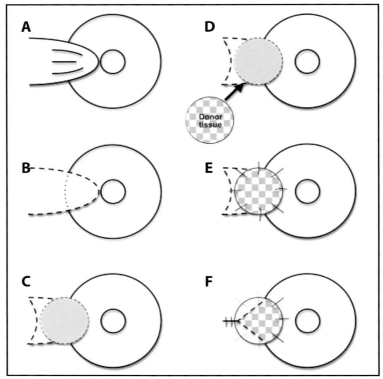

Figure 2-5. Excision of pterygium and placement of lamellar corneoscleral graft. (A) Large nasal pterygium. (B) Pterygium excised from cornea and adjacent anterior nasal sclera. (C) A penetrating keratoplasty trephine is used to perform a partial (not full) thickness circular incision involving the peripheral cornea and adjacent anterior sclera. A partial-thickness lamellar dissection is then performed in the shaded gray area encompassed by the partial-thickness circular trephine incision. The lamellar dissection performed in the circular gray area creates a recipient bed for donor corneal tissue. (D) Donor corneal tissue is prepared using a corneal trephine with approximately the same diameter used to outline the lamellar recipient bed created by lamellar dissection described in the preceding illustration (see Figure 2-4C). (E) Donor corneal tissue is placed in the corneoscleral recipient bed, and secured with multiple interrupted sutures. (F) Adjacent normal conjunctiva may be mobilized and re-positioned to partially cover the scleral portion of the donor corneal graft tissue. (Illustration created by Vicky C. Pai, MD and Mr. Chuck Feldman.)

Conclusion

This chapter has reviewed the evolution of pterygium surgery, from the distant past through the latter part of the 20th century. The older techniques all suffered from high rates of recurrence; many of the early techniques also caused other very significant complications. The more modern techniques described elsewhere in this textbook have either been proven, or hold great promise, to significantly improve the management of this common, troublesome, and sometimes very difficult disorder.

References

1. Hirschberg J, Blodi FC, Heitz RF. *The History of Ophthalmology.* Vol 1. Bonn, Germany: J.P. Wayenborgh; 1982:238-239.
2. Hirschberg J, Blodi FC, Heitz RF. *The History of Ophthalmology.* Vol 2. Bonn, Germany: J.P. Wayenborgh; 1982:333-334.
3. Buratto L, Phillips RL, Carito G. *Pterygium Surgery.* Thorofare, NJ: SLACK Incorporated; 2000:5.
4. Fuchs E. *Text-Book of Ophthalmology.* New York, NY: D. Appleton & Company; 1893.
5. Riordan-Eva P, Kielhorn I, Ficker LA, Steele AD, Kirkness CM. Conjunctival autografting in the surgical management of pterygium. *Eye (Lond).* 1993;7(Pt 5):634-638.
6. McReynolds JO. The nature and treatment of pterygia. *JAMA.* 1902;39(6):296-299.
7. Neher EM. A new method of transplanting pterygium. *Trans Am Ophthalmol Soc.* 1938;36:163-170.
8. Knapp H. New plastic conjunctival operation. *Arch Ophthalmol.* 1868;14:270-272.
9. Rosen E. Pterygium. *Br J Ophthalmol.* 1948;32(5):300-304.
10. Kamel S. Pterygium. Its nature and a new line of treatment. *Br J Ophthalmol.* 1946;30(9):549-563.
11. D'Ombrain A. The surgical treatment of pterygium. *Br J Ophthalmol.* 1948;32(2):65-71.
12. King JH. The pterygium; brief review and evaluation of certain methods of treatment. *Arch Ophthalmol.* 1950;44(6):854-869.
13. McGavic JS. Surgical treatment of recurrent pterygium. *Arch Ophthalmol.* 1949;42(6):726-748.
14. Singh G, Wilson MR, Foster CS. Mitomycin eye drops as treatment for pterygium. *Ophthalmology.* 1988;95(6):813-821.
15. Tan DT, Chee SP, Dear KB, Lim AS. Effect of pterygium morphology on pterygium recurrence in a controlled trial comparing conjunctival autografting with bare sclera excision. *Arch Ophthalmol.* 1997;115(10):1235-1240.
16. Iliff CE. Beta irradiation in ophthalmology. *Am J Ophthalmol.* 1948;31(3):339.
17. Friedell HL, Thomas CI, Krohmer JS. Description of an Sr-90 beta-ray applicator and its use on the eye. *Am J Roentgenol Radium Ther.* 1951;65(2):232-244.
18. Rosenthal JW. Beta-radiation therapy of pterygium. *AMA Arch Ophthalmol.* 1953;49(1):17-23.
19. Kirwan JF, Constable PH, Murdoch IE, Khaw PT. Beta irradiation: new uses for an old treatment: a review. *Eye (Lond).* 2003;17(2):207-215.
20. Campbell OR, Amendola BE, Brady LW. Recurrent pterygia: results of postoperative treatment with Sr-90 applicators. *Radiology.* 1990;174(2):565-566.
21. Brenner DJ, Merriam GR, Jr. Postoperative irradiation for pterygium: guidelines for optimal treatment. *Int J Radiat Oncol Biol Phys.* 1994;30(3):721-725.
22. Hirst LW. The treatment of pterygium. *Surv Ophthalmol.* 2003;48(2):145-180.
23. Paryani SB, Scott WP, Wells JW, Jr., et al. Management of pterygium with surgery and radiation therapy. The North Florida Pterygium Study Group. *Int J Radiat Oncol Biol Phys.* 1994;28(1):101-103.
24. Mourits MP, Wyrdeman HK, Jurgenliemk-Schulz IM, Bidlot E. Favorable long-term results of primary pterygium removal by bare sclera extirpation followed by a single 90Strontium application. *Eur J Ophthalmol.* 2008;18(3):327-331.
25. Altman AJ, Cohen EJ, Berger ST, Mondino BJ. Scleritis and *Streptococcus pneumoniae. Cornea.* 1991;10(4):341-345.
26. Farrell PL, Smith RE. Bacterial corneoscleritis complicating pterygium excision. *Am J Ophthalmol.* 1989;107(5):515-517.
27. MacKenzie FD, Hirst LW, Kynaston B, Bain C. Recurrence rate and complications after beta irradiation for pterygia. *Ophthalmology.* 1991;98(12):1776-1780; discussion 1781.
28. Tarr KH, Constable IJ. Late complications of pterygium treatment. *Br J Ophthalmol.* 1980;64(7):496-505.
29. Ngoy D, Kayembe L. [A comparative study of thio-tepa and mitomycin C in the treatment of pterygium. Preliminary results]. *J Fr Ophtalmol.* 1998;21(2):96-102.
30. Tassy A, Ribe D. [Thiotepa eyedrops for prevention of pterygium recurrence: 18 years of use]. *J Fr Ophtalmol.* 1999;22(2):215-219.
31. Klein S. Zur operation des pterygium und zur transplantation vom schleimhaut. *Allg. Wein. med. Ztg.* 1876;21:19.
32. Elschnig HH. A new operation for replapsing pterygium. *Klin. Monatsbl. f. Augenh.* 1926;76:714.
33. Gomez-Maequez J. New operative procedure for pterygium. *Arch de oftal. Hispano-am.* 1931;31:87.
34. Thoft RA. Conjunctival transplantation. *Arch Ophthalmol.* 1977;95(8):1425-1427.
35. Kenyon KR, Wagoner MD, Hettinger ME. Conjunctival autograft transplantation for advanced and recurrent pterygium. *Ophthalmology.* 1985;92(11):1461-1470.

36. Hotz FC. A few experiments with Thiersch grafts in the operation of pterygium. *JAMA.* 1892;19:297.
37. Gifford H. Treatment of recurrent pterygium. *Ophthalmol Rec.* 1909;18:1.
38. Magitot A. A critical study of certain biological properties of the corneal tissue and of human keratoplasty. *Ann. d'Ocul.* 1916;152:417.
39. Reeh MJ. Corneoscleral lamellar transplant for recurrent pterygium. *Arch Ophthalmol.* 1971;86(3):296-297.
40. Reis JL. A corneal graft operation for recurrent pterygium. *Brit J Ophthalmol.* 1945;29:637.
41. Suveges I. Sclerokeratoplasty in recurrent pterygium. *Ger J Ophthalmol.* 1992;1(2):114-116.
42. Panzardi D. Use of fetal membranes as material for plastic restoration of conjunctiva, with special regard to their use in pterygium. *Boll. d'Ocul.* 1947;26:332.

3

Pterygium Excision With Conjunctival Autograft

Kenneth R. Kenyon, MD and Mark A. Fava, MD, FRCSC

Pterygium excision with conjunctival autograft transplantation remains the procedure of choice for definitive treatment of both primary and recurrent pterygia. By replacing the area of pterygium-altered conjunctiva with normal bulbar conjunctival tissue, this technically straightforward surgical technique has long been proven to be efficacious with respect to minimal pterygium recurrence and long-term safety.[1,2] The basic technique, as originally devised in the 1980s,[1,3-5] has subsequently been modified to include the use of tissue adhesives[6-10] and adjunctive antimetabolite treatment.[11-15]

Historical reviews of pterygium surgery include such archaic approaches as bare sclera excision, burying the head of the pterygium, mucus membrane, and even skin grafts; laser ablation; and adjunctive use of beta irradiation,[16] thiotepa,[17,18] and mitomycin-C (MMC).[11-15] Regrettably, all such strategies are subject to either unacceptably high recurrence rates (60% or more) and/or wound healing complications such as avascular scleral necrosis (Figure 3-1A).[19-25] Other useful approaches including primary conjunctival closure,[26] rotational flaps,[27] and variations of Z-plasty may be effective but are beyond the scope of this discussion. The use of either frozen or lyophilized human amniotic membrane transplantation (AMT)[28,29] for this purpose has also been promoted, and this important application will also be subsequently discussed.

Definitive surgical treatment is appropriately indicated when—despite conservative medical management—the pterygium either reduces vision by progressively encroaching upon the corneal visual axis or inducing corneal astigmatism and/or by stimulating chronic ocular irritation and inflammation. Indeed, the medical treatment of pterygia is traditionally conservative, designed to decrease irritative symptoms, to reduce conjunctival tissue swelling and inflammation, and to slow progression. Tear function testing (Schirmer), lid closure, and blink adequacy must be assessed to rule out associated intrinsic dry eye and exposure components. Topical therapy can then consist of artificial tears, lubricants, vasoconstrictors, anti-histamines (including naphazoline, olopatadine, epinastine), nonsteroidal anti-inflammatory drugs (NSAIDs; such as ketorolac), and corticosteroids (ranging from fluorometholone to prednisolone or dexamethasone). Use of ultra violet (UV)-blocking sunglasses and broad-brimmed hats

Hovanesian JA. *Pterygium: Techniques and Technologies for Surgical Success (pp 37-48)*
© 2012 Taylor & Francis Group

Figure 3-1. Surgical complications. (A) Avascular scleral necrosis caused by prolonged MMC application following pterygium excision without conjunctival autograft transplantation. (B) Hypertrophic pedunculated focal pyogenic granuloma following conjunctival autograft.

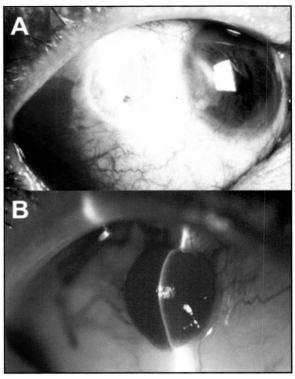

plus reduction in environmental exposures may also reduce inflammatory episodes and progression. In the absence of a truly aqueous deficient dry eye, neither punctum occlusion nor topical cyclosporine (Restasis) appear to be beneficial.

The indications for surgical intervention then include chronic inflammation and/or irritation of cosmetic consequence, not relieved by the above specified medical therapy; documented progression to threaten visual axis; and decreased vision due to either visual axis involvement and/or induced astigmatism.

Surgical Management of Pterygium

Preferred Surgical Technique

Once the aforementioned surgical indications are met, we believe there is no need to hesitate or to vary the surgical technique of conjunctival autograft transplantation as developed at the Massachusetts Eye & Ear Infirmary in the early 1980s, extending on Thoft's earlier work in conjunctival autografting (albeit then largely for uniocular chemical injuries). Coincidentally and entirely unbeknownst to us at the time, the great Professor Jose Barraquer had briefly described a very similar method in the proceedings of the World Cornea Congress as early as 1964! The basic technique remains largely unaltered as described in our original series,[1] save for the relatively recent utilization of fibrin tissue adhesive (eg, Tisseel, Baxter Healthcare Corp, Deerfield, IL; Figures 3-2C and 3-2D).

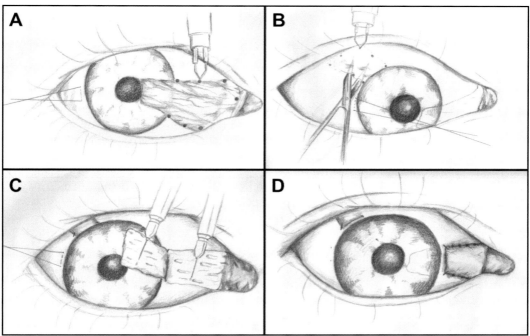

Figure 3-2. (A) Conjunctival autograft surgical technique. A limbal traction suture (8-0 Vicryl) externally rotates the eye to maximally expose the pterygium. A disposable low-temp cautery is used to delineate the area of conjunctiva, including the semi-lunar fold, to be excised. (B) Following pterygium excision, the eye is rotated down and in to expose the superior temporal bulbar conjunctiva. Cautery spots are again utilized to define the exact area of the conjunctival autograft. Westcott scissors are used to blunt dissect conjunctiva as thinly as possible from the underlying Tenon's tissue, and then the graft is excised to retain the cautery marks within the graft margins to assist with proper orientation and positioning at the transplantation site. The donor site is closed with a single diagonal suture of 8-0 Vicryl. (C) The conjunctival graft is appropriately positioned in the exposed scleral bed. If desired, 2 Vicryl sutures are placed to properly secure the medial margins 1 to 2 mm posterior to the limbus. The graft is then turned centrally to overlie the cornea, thereby exposing the stromal surface of the graft so that the more viscous sealer protein plus aprotinin component of the fibrin adhesive can be applied to the graft stroma, while the less viscous thrombin component is applied over the sclera and rectus muscle. (Prior to conjunctival graft adhesion and if necessary to obtain adequate hemostasis, fibrin adhesive can also be applied into the depth of the medial fornix.) (D) The conjunctival graft is turned and held in position to cover the entire scleral bed. If apposition to close the defect between the graft margin and caruncle is not adequate, then additional 8-0 Vicryl sutures can be placed, as this closure is important to prevent recurrence.

The technique and comments on specific steps are as follows (Figure 3-2):

1. Anesthesia is either topical tetracaine +/- subconjunctival xylocaine for primary pterygia; however, peri- or retrobulbar xylocaine/marcaine is preferable for advanced primary or recurrent cases, especially if the latter involve fibrosis of the subjacent rectus muscle causing mechanical extraocular movement restriction and hence requiring extensive surgical manipulation and dissection.

2. A limbal traction suture (8-0 Vicryl, Ethicon, Inc, Somerville, NJ) is placed at the opposite limbus (eg, temporal if pterygium nasal), and the globe is rotated to maximally expose the pterygium (Figure 3-2A).

3. Using a disposable low-temperature cautery, 6 to 8 spots are placed to delineate the body of the pterygium and adjacent tissue (often including the semilunar fold)

to be excised. This is of great benefit because the surgeon can literally "connect the dots" and be certain that exactly the appropriate tissue has been removed.

4. Grasping the pterygium head with 0.3 Castroviejo forceps, the cap is then dissected by probing with dry surgical sponges (Weck-cel, Medtronic, Minneapolis, MN), scraping with a crescent or scarifier (Beaver 57, Beaver Visitec International, Waltham, MA) blade held perpendicularly to the corneal surface and then avulsing and/or stripping the corneal portion solely by blunt technique, as would be appropriate for superficial keratectomy. As the pterygium invariably advances over the corneal surface, incision into the stroma is never necessary or appropriate, as the resultant stromal thinning may increase the likelihood of dellen formation or even require sectoral lamellar keratoplasty. Superficial and blunt dissection entirely avoids this potential complication. It is important to smooth the surface of the cornea and adjacent limbus by rapid stroking/scraping with the perpendicularly oriented scarifier blade. Alternatively, a manual or motorized diamond burr may also be utilized.

5. Undermine the body with spring-action Westcott scissors, constantly seeking the subjacent rectus muscle. Especially in recurrent cases, this muscle becomes enmeshed in scar tissue which not only limits its action (causing extraocular movement [EOM] restriction) but also disguises its identity, placing it at risk to be damaged or even severed unless extreme caution is exercised in appropriate identification and isolation (as with traction suture or muscle hook). Only when clearly identified and cleanly dissected can the adjacent conjunctiva, Tenon's tissue, and scar tissue be excised without risk. Once this is accomplished, and especially in EOM-restricted cases, the rectus must be freed of all associated connective tissue such that the adjacent and subjacent sclera is bare.

6. In approaching the medial canthus while dissecting prolapsed orbital fat, caution must be exercised to avoid severing blood vessels, which can be extremely difficult to cauterize. Should deep bleeders that defy visualization and cauterization be encountered, cut the triangular head from a cellulose surgical sponge and stuff this into the recess between the rectus and the plica. The bleeding will cease and definitive hemostasis can subsequently be obtained by rapidly withdrawing the sponge and dripping the 2-part fibrin glue into the depth of the wound to produce an adhesive seal.

7. Once the bare scleral area is defined, measure the resultant conjunctival defect with calipers. The use of MMC 0.02% is rarely required in more than 5% of cases but should be considered in specific instances (eg, when a previously well performed conjunctival autograft has failed with recurrence or when an extremely inflamed pterygium in a high recurrence risk patient is encountered). In these situations, small surgical sponge segments are soaked in MMC and placed in the fornix recesses beneath the cut margins of the conjunctiva, avoiding exposure to the bare sclera and rectus muscle. After 3 minutes, the sponges are removed, and the surgical field is copiously irrigated with at least 15 mL of balanced salt solution (BSS).

8. To prepare the conjunctival autograft, turn the globe down and in with the traction suture, thereby exposing the superotemporal bulbar conjunctiva (see Figure 3-2B). Using the calipers, measure an area on the conjunctival surface sufficient to cover the exposed sclera and rectus muscle, and mark the perimeter with approximately 6 cautery spots. Be generous—there is no need to undersize the autograft as the conjunctiva here is extremely redundant, and grafts as large as 10 x 15 mm will

consistently vascularize without risk of ischemia. Excise the graft using Westcott scissors, first performing a radial conjunctival incision, then undermining bluntly to separate conjunctiva from Tenon's tissue, and finally completing excision such that all cautery marks remain within the margins of the graft. Injection of minimal anesthetic or BSS into the donor conjunctival area to "balloon" the tissue may be helpful, but careful blunt dissection with spring-action scissors is preferable to obtain a graft as thin as possible. The retention of the cautery marks is absolutely key to assist in spreading and orienting the graft correctly and especially in avoiding any "down-side risk" of inversion. After obtaining hemostasis in the donor site, close the donor site with a single 8-0 Vicryl suture, which diagonally spans the conjunctival defect.

9. Return the eye to maximal abduction and orient the autograft in its corresponding position to cover the exposed sclera. The corneal edge of the graft should be 1 mm posterior to the limbus, and two 8-0 Vicryl sutures may be optionally placed to secure the central margin of the graft in this position. The peripheral margin of the graft is then grasped with 2 forceps and is reflected to overlie the cornea with its stromal surface exposed. The 2 fibrin adhesive components are then applied, with the more viscous sealer protein plus aprotinin on the graft stromal surface and the thinner thrombin on the bare sclera "peanut butter and jelly sandwich style," as described by Eliot Perlman, MD (personal communication, 2000; see Figure 3-2C). The free edges of the graft are again grasped with forceps, and the tissue is again inverted to "sandwich" the exposed sclera and thereby establish the adhesive bond, which is accomplished within 30 seconds. If the graft is adequately sized and the margins are well apposed to the adjacent conjunctiva, especially at the plica, then the procedure is complete (see Figure 3-2D). However, if there is a persistent gap, then additional 8-0 Vicryl sutures will be needed to secure the corners of the graft. (Note: If fibrin adhesive is not available or affordable, then the conjunctival graft can be entirely secured with a total of 6 sutures of 8-0 Vicryl, representing less than 5 minutes of additional operating time and a savings of approximately $150. Though some surgeons prefer 10-0 nylon sutures, our preference remains Vicryl since it is nearly nonreactive and its absorbability saves significant office time and patient angst over suture removal).

10. The limbal traction suture is then removed and, especially if the corneal epithelial defect is extensive, a standard size bandage soft contact lens is applied along with topical antibiotic, corticosteroid, and NSAID, plus or minus a semi-pressure patch until the first postoperative visit. Adequate systemic analgesia (eg, acetaminophen, oxycodone [Percocet] 5/325 mg or acetaminophen [Tylenol] plus codeine 30 mg) should be provided for the first 24 to 48 hours.

Variations for Special Situations

For recurrent pterygia, if the previous procedure did not involve conjunctival autograft transplantation, then—having waited at least 3 months following the most recent surgery and having utilized topical steroids to dissipate inflammation—a standard conjunctival autograft is performed (Figures 3-3 and 3-4). If the prior surgery did comprise conjunctival autografting, then the recommended approach is a repeat conjunctival autograft with MMC 0.02% intraoperatively as previously described. For simultaneous nasal and temporal pterygia, the standard procedure is performed identically at both sites of involvement utilizing donor grafts from either superiorly and inferiorly of the same eye and/or harvesting one of the grafts from the fellow eye. This poses

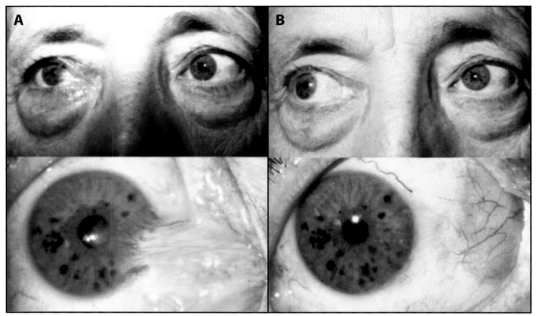

Figure 3-3. Recurrent pterygium in a 64-year-old man who had undergone 5 previous pterygium excisions in his right eye. (A) Top: There is marked restriction of right abduction with clinically significant diplopia. Bottom: A dense band of scar tissue obliterates the medial fornix and displaces the caruncle nearly to the limbus. (B) Top: More than 4 years after conjunctival autograft transplantation, extraocular movements are full, as right abduction is unrestricted. Bottom: The operated eye is uninflamed, and the pterygium has not recurred. (Reprinted with permission from *Ophthalmology*, 92(11), Kenyon KR, Wagoner MD, Hettinger ME, Conjunctival autograft transplantation for advanced and recurrent pterygium, 1461-1470, Copyright Elsevier (1985).)

no risk whatsoever of "donor depletion." The bulbar conjunctiva is abundant and has little tendency to scar or form symblepharon when harvested properly and does not involve limbal stem cell expenditure, as the limbal tissue is altogether spared in the donor preparation. Thus it is only the extremely rare circumstance where such extensive fornix reconstruction in conjunction with pterygium excision must be performed as to warrant the use of AMT.

Postoperative Therapy

The typical "triple therapy" of a fluoroquinolone antibiotic, NSAID, and corticosteroid is initiated 4 times daily, but if inflammation is not abating at 1 week follow-up, then the steroid dose is increased to every 1 or 2 hours. The antibiotic and NSAID are usually discontinued at 1 week, and the steroids are titrated according to the degree of inflammation over a 1 month interval at least, but often with continuation for 2 or occasionally 3 months. Steroids should not be discontinued either prematurely or arbitrarily, as rebound inflammation can be substantial. If excessive inflammation persists at 1 month, then subconjunctival triamcinolone (Kenalog) 0.3 mL is injected adjacent to the grafted area. As long as "strong" steroids are in use, intraocular pressure and lens clarity must be closely monitored. The bandage soft contact lens is removed usually between 2 to 5 days or as soon as the corneal epithelial defect has healed. Systemic analgesia is seldom required for more than 1 week. UV-blocking sunglasses are recommended for continuous and life-long outdoor use.

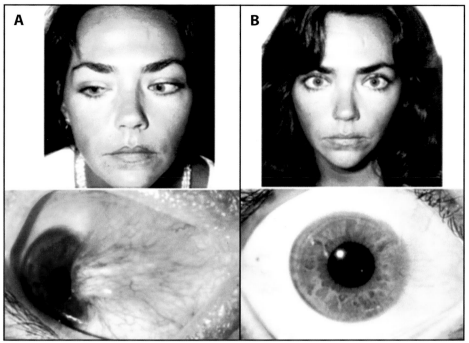

Figure 3-4. Recurrent pterygium in a 29-year-old woman with 2 previous surgical failures. (A) Top: Diplopia upon attempted right gaze due to mechanical cicatricial restriction. Bottom: The recurrent pterygium is fleshy and inflamed. (B) Top: Three months following conjunctival autograft transplantation, the cosmetic and symptomatic improvement is excellent. Bottom: The operated eye is uninflamed and there is no limitation of movement. Follow-up in this case is currently more than 15 years without recurrence. (Reprinted with permission from *Ophthalmology*, 92(11), Kenyon KR, Wagoner MD, Hettinger ME, Conjunctival autograft transplantation for advanced and recurrent pterygium, 1461-1470, Copyright Elsevier (1985).)

Complications

Conjunctival grafts never fail, and even minor complications are extremely uncommon. If the corneal margin of the graft is correctly placed 1 to 2 mm posterior to the limbus, then corneal dellen are unusual and are self-resolving with increased lubricants and large diameter soft contact lenses. Unless the graft is mechanically displaced (in which case it can be repositioned and secured with 8-0 Vicryl) or lost (an extremely rare event), avascular persistent epithelial defects of the exposed sclera are exceedingly seldom, and avascular stromalysis of the sclera occurs only in situations where excessive or misapplied MMC had been utilized (see Figure 3-1A). Hypertrophic fibrovascular pyogenic granulomas (see Figure 3-1B) seldom occur and usually "dissolve" spontaneously with topical steroids or, as they are usually pedunculated, can be simply excised with a single snip at the slit-lamp.

Outcomes

The encouraging results of our initial series[1] of predominantly recurrent cases comprised 95% success (ie, no recurrence and cosmetically acceptable; Figure 3-5) with 100% motility improvement in eyes with restrictive strabismus. This outcome has remained our consistent result over the ensuing 25 years and has been confirmed in published comparative series by many authors internationally.[1-3,29-36]

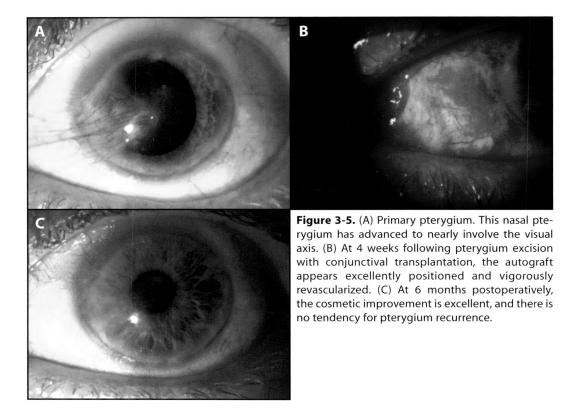

Figure 3-5. (A) Primary pterygium. This nasal pterygium has advanced to nearly involve the visual axis. (B) At 4 weeks following pterygium excision with conjunctival transplantation, the autograft appears excellently positioned and vigorously revascularized. (C) At 6 months postoperatively, the cosmetic improvement is excellent, and there is no tendency for pterygium recurrence.

Most importantly, the pterygium recurrence rate is less than 5%, even in previously recurrent cases involving cicatricial strabismus (see Figures 3-3 and 3-4). To date, we are unaware of any report utilizing alternative (eg, AMT) or adjunctive (eg, MMC) techniques, which have shown superior outcomes in any respect.[29-36] Moreover, for the more challenging cases of recurrent pterygia with motility restriction, excessive scarring, and exaggerated inflammation, conjunctival grafting clearly remains superior.

Alternative Techniques and the Evolution of the Conjunctival Autograft

Surgical management of pterygia continues to evolve. However, the preferred surgical strategy for primary cases, and especially for the more challenging situations posed by recurrent pterygia, almost certainly remains conjunctival autograft transplantation. Whatever the surgical variation, the fundamental procedure remains to be the transfer of a conjunctival autograft to cover the conjunctival defect and bare sclera exposed by the pterygium excision.

Such surgical variations include small excision, the mini-flap technique,[37] narrow-strip excision,[38] mini-autografting,[39] sliding flap,[40] rotational autograft,[27,41] and extended excisions.[42] These techniques have all shown good efficacy with respect to recurrence and complications since they are all based on the axiom of replacing the excised area with an autograft.

The 2 most studied adjunctive therapies that have become appropriately integrated into the basic conjunctival autograft technique are intraoperative application of MMC[33-35,43] and the use of tissue adhesives.[29,44,45] With or without these additional measures, the conjunctival autograft technique remains superior to any comparative surgical technique with respect to recurrence and complications.

AMT treatment is another variation on this theme but has not been shown to be superior to conjunctival autografting.[29,32,36,46] With respect to AMT in particular, the addition of 5 minutes of surgical time for conjunctival graft preparation does not justify, in our view, the additional expense (which costs at least $500 in the United States) and logistical effort of obtaining the tissue. To be sure, we remain major enthusiasts of AMT. Considering the ability of inlay grafts to heal persistent corneal epithelial defects and ulcers and for overlay grafts to promote limbal stem cell transplantation, fornix reconstruction, and neurotrophic keratoplasty, AMT gives the surgeon another option when conjunctiva is in short supply or in the rare event that glaucoma filtering surgery may be involved. Having reviewed the evidence for this position relatively recently, our stated position remains unaltered.[28]

Conclusion

Although alternative and adjunctive approaches including amnion membrane transplantation and MMC are applicable, the basic conjunctival autograft technique—now further simplified and nearly sutureless since the advent of fibrin adhesives—remains the safe, effective, and economical procedure of choice. Above all, please remember that as a substitute for conjunctiva, there simply remains nothing better than conjunctiva.

References

1. Kenyon KR, Wagoner MD, Hettinger ME. Conjunctival autograft transplantation for advanced and recurrent pterygium. *Ophthalmology*. 1985;92:1461-1470.
2. Allan BD, Short P, Crawford GJ, et al. Pterygium excision with conjunctival autografting: an effective and safe technique. *Br J Ophthalmol*. 1993;77:698-701.
3. Starck, T, Kenyon, KR, Serrano F. Conjunctival autograft for primary and recurrent pterygia: surgical technique and problem management. *Cornea*. 1991;10(3):196-202.
4. Hirst LW. The treatment of pterygium. *Surv Ophthalmol*. 2003;48:145-180.
5. Ang LP, Chua JL, Tan DT. Current concepts and techniques in pterygium treatment. *Curr Opin Ophthalmol*. 2007;18:308-313.
6. Koranyi G, Seregard S, Kopp ED. Cut and paste: a no suture, small incision approach to pterygium surgery. *Br J Ophthalmol*. 2004;88:911-914.
7. Koranyi G, Seregard S, Kopp ED. The cut-and-paste method for primary surgery: long-term follow-up. *Acta Ophthalmol Scand*. 2005;83:298-301.
8. Marticorena J, Rodruguez-Ares MT, Tourino R, et al. Pterygium surgery: conjunctival autograft using a fibrin adhesive. *Cornea*. 2006;25:34-36.
9. Uy HS, Reyes JM, Flores JD, et al. Comparison of fibrin glue and sutures for attaching conjunctival autografts after pterygium excision. *Ophthalmology*. 2005;112:667-671.
10. Bahar I, Weinberger D, Gaton DD, et al. Fibrin glue versus vicryl sutures for primary conjunctival closure in pterygium surgery: long-term results. *Curr Eye Res*. 2007;32:399-405.
11. Cano-Parra J, Diaz-Llopis M, Maldonado MJ, et al. Prospective trial of intraoperative mitomycin C in the treatment of primary pterygium. *Br J Ophthalmol*. 1995;79:439-441.
12. Frucht-Pery J, Charalambos SS, Ilsar M. Intraoperative application of topical mitomycin C for pterygium surgery. *Ophthalmology*. 1996;103:674-677.

13. Lam DS, Wong AK, Fan DS, et al. Intraoperative mitomycin C to prevent recurrence of pterygium after excision: a 30-month follow-up study. *Ophthalmology.* 1998;105:901-904.
14. Manning CA, Kloess PM, Diaz MD, Yee RW. Intraoperative mitomycin in primary pterygium excision: a prospective, randomized trial. *Ophthalmology.* 1997;104:844-848.
15. Raiskup F, Solomon A, Landau D, et al. Mitomycin C for pterygium: long term evaluation. *Br J Ophthalmol.* 2004;88:1425-1428.
16. Alaniz-Camino F. The use of postoperative beta radiation in the treatment of pterygia. *Ophthalmic Surg.* 1982;12:1022-1025.
17. Cassady JR. The inhibition of pterygium recurrence by thio-tepa. *Am K Ophthalmol.* 1966;61:886-887.
18. Asregadoo ER. Surgery, thio-tepa, and corticosteroid in the treatment of pterygium. *Am J Ophthalmol.* 1972;74:960-963.
19. Alsagoff Z, Tan DT, Chee SP. Necrotising scleritis after bare sclera excision of pterygium. *Br J Ophthalmol.* 2000;84(9):1050-1052.
20. Cappin JM: Radiation scleral necrosis simulating early scleromalacia perforans. *Br J Ophthalmol.* 1973;57:425-8.
21. Rubinfeld RS, Pfister RR, Stein RM, et al. Serious complications of topical mitomycin-C after pterygium surgery. *Ophthalmology.* 1992;99:1647-1654.
22. Moriarty AP, Crawford GJ, McAllister IL, Constable IJ. Severe corneoscleral infection: a complication of beta irradiation scleral necrosis following pterygium excision. *Arch Ophthalmol.* 1993;11:947-951.
23. Dunn JP, Seamone CD, Ostler HB, et al. Development of scleral ulceration and calcification after pterygium excision and mitomycin therapy. *Am J Ophthalmol.* 1991;112:343-344.
24. Dougherty PJ, Hardten DR, Lindstrom RL. Corneoscleral melt after pterygium surgery using a single intraoperative application of mitomycin-C. *Cornea.* 1996;15:537-540.
25. Dusenbery KE, Alul IH, Holland EJ, et al. Beta irradiation of recurrent pterygia: results and complications. *Int J Radiat Oncol Biol Phys.* 1992;24:315-320.
26. Prabhasawat P, Barton K, Burkett G, Tseng SC. Comparison of conjunctival autografts, amniotic membrane grafts, and primary closure for pterygium excision. *Ophthalmology.* 1997;104(6):974-85.
27. Jap A, Chan C, Lim L, Tan DT. Conjunctival autorotation autograft for pterygium: an alternative to conjunctival autografting. *Ophthalmology.* 1999;106:67-71.
28. Kenyon KR. Amniotic membrane: mother's own remedy for ocular surface disease. *Cornea.* 2005;24(6):639-642.
29. Luanratanakorn P, Ratanapakorn T, Suwan-Apichon O, Chuck RS. Randomized controlled study of conjunctival autograft versus amniotic membrane graft in pterygium excision. *Br J Ophthalmol.* 2006;90:1476-1480.
30. Katircioglu YA, Altiparmak UE, Duman S. Comparison of three methods for the treatment of pterygium: amniotic membrane graft, conjunctival autograft and conjunctival autograft plus mitomycin C. *Orbit.* 2007;26(1):5-13.
31. Kuzmanovic Elabjer B, Busic M, Elabjar, E. Retrospective clinical analysis of free conjunctival autograft in treatment of pterygia. *Collegium Antropologicum.* 2008;32(1):303-306.
32. Kucukerdonmez C, Akova YA, Altinors DD. Comparison of conjunctival autograft with amniotic membrane transplantation for pterygium surgery: surgical and cosmetic outcome. *Cornea.* 2007;26(4):407-413.
33. Akinci A, Zilelioglu O. Comparison of limbal-conjunctival autograft and intraoperative 0.02% mitomycin-C for treatment of primary pterygium. *In Ophthalmol.* 2007;27:281-285.
34. Biswas MC, Shaw C, Mandel R, et al. Treatment of pterygium with conjunctival limbal autograft and mitomycin C: a comparative study. *J Indian Med Assoc.* 2007;105:200,202,204.
35. Young AL, Leung GY, Wong AK, et al. A randomized trial comparing 0.02% mitomycin C and limbal conjunctival autograft after excision of primary pterygium. *Br J Ophthalmol.* 2004;88:995-997.
36. Tananuvat N, Martin T. The results of amniotic membrane transplantation for primary pterygium compared with conjunctival autograft. *Cornea.* 2004;23:458-463.
37. Kim M, Chung SH, Lee JH, Lee HK, Seo KY. Comparison of mini-flap technique and conjunctival autograft transplantation without mitomycin C in primary and recurrent pterygium. *Ophthalmologica;* 2008;222(4):265-271.
38. Dupps WJ Jr., Jeng BH, Meisler DM. Narrow-strip conjunctival autograft for treatment of pterygium. *Ophthalmology.* 2006;114:227-231.
39. Oguz H, Kilitcioglu A, Yasar M. Limbal conjunctival mini-autografting for preventing recurrence after pterygium surgery. *Eur J Ophthalmol.* 2006;16:209-213.
40. Tomas T. Sliding flap of conjunctival limbus to prevent recurrence of pterygium. *Refract Corneal Surg.* 1992;8:394-395.
41. Dadeya S, Malik KP, Gullian BP. Pterygium surgery: conjunctival rotation autograft versus conjunctival autograft. *Ophthalmic Surg Lasers.* 2002;33:269-274.

42. Hirst LW. Recurrent pterygium surgery using pterygium extended removal followed by extended conjunctival transplant: recurrence rate and cosmesis. *Ophthalmology.* 2009;116(7):1278-1286.
43. Altiparmak UE, Katircioglu YA, Yagci R, Yalniz Z, Duman S. Mitomycin C and conjunctival autograft for recurrent pterygium. *International Ophthalmology.* 2007;27(6):339-343.
44. Hall RC, Logan AJ, Wells AP. Comparison of fibrin glue with sutures for pterygium excision with conjunctival autografts. *Clinical & Experimental Ophthalmology.* 2009;37(6):584-589.
45. Srinivasan S, Dollin M, McAllum P, Berger Y, Rootman DS, Slomovic AR. Fibrin glue versus sutures for attaching the conjunctival autograft in pterygium surgery: a prospective observer masked clinical trial. *Br J Ophthalmol.* 2009;93(2):215-218.
46. Ozer A, Yildirim N, Erol N, Yurdakul S. Long-term results of bare sclera, limbal-conjunctival autograft and amniotic membrane graft techniques in primary pterygium excisions. *Ophthalmologica.* 2009; 223(4):269-273.

4

Fibrin Tissue Adhesive

David R. Hardten, MD

Fibrin sealants have been used for more than 20 years, primarily as an adjunct to hemostasis in cardiovascular surgery and trauma.[1,2] The first reported use was for skin graft fixation in 1944.[3] Around that same time, it was used in experiments fixating corneal grafts in rabbits.[4] Fibrin sealant was approved by the United States Food and Drug Administration (FDA) in May 1998. At this point, no fibrin adhesive has been approved for use in ophthalmology, although it is widely used in an off-label fashion mainly because suturing is time consuming, and sutures may cause tissue reaction and inflammation. Despite the development of other adhesives, those based on the coagulation cascade are still most commonly utilized.

A major advantage of fibrin adhesive is that it allows sufficient working time before it obtains final firm adhesion. It also has adequate strength to maintain wound integrity, especially against sliding forces, which is very helpful for conjunctival and corneal applications. It does not induce significant inflammation and is also slowly resorbed so that it does not risk pulling the tissues apart when it completes its useful wound healing. Because it is commonly used in other applications such as abdominal and thoracic surgery, it is readily available in almost any hospital or outpatient surgical system. Some forms of fibrin sealant are available at room temperature, while some are preserved in a cool environment.

Mechanism of Action

Fibrin glue imitates the final stages of the coagulation cascade when fibrinogen is activated by thrombin. The adhesive capacity of the fibrin glue mimics the coagulation cascade.[5-7] During the coagulation cascade, factor X is activated and selectively hydrolyses prothrombin to thrombin. In the presence of thrombin, fibrinogen is converted to fibrin. Factor XIII, which is present in the fibrinogen component of the glue, is also activated by the thrombin. The factor XIII promotes polymerization and cross linking of the fibrin chains to stabilize the clot by forming long fibrin strands, assisted by the presence of calcium. The fibrin clot degrades gradually over a few weeks.

Hovanesian JA. *Pterygium: Techniques and Technologies for Surgical Success (pp 49-54)*
© 2012 Taylor & Francis Group

Fibrin sealant is composed of 2 main components: a sealer protein concentrate that contains fibrinogen and a fibrinolysis inhibitor as well as a thrombin and calcium chloride solution.[8] These 2 solutions are kept separate until the time of the procedure. When they are mixed, they mimic the human clotting cascade. The 2 components are mixed at the tip of a double-barreled syringe, or they can be applied individually by separate syringes and mixed on the target tissue to create adhesion. Once the 2 solutions come into contact with each other, the surgeon has between 10 and 60 seconds to manipulate the glue, depending on the thrombin concentration.

Formulations Available

Several companies make fibrin sealant, but only 2 companies produce fibrin sealant that is available in the United States. Baxter Healthcare Corp (Deerfield, IL) makes Tisseel and Artiss, and Ethicon, Inc (Somerville, NJ) makes Evicel.

Tisseel fibrin sealant is approved by the FDA. It comes as a 2-component product, stored at room temperature in the freeze-dried form, or is also available as frozen prefilled syringes. In the vapor heated (VH) form, the blue bottle is a sealer protein concentrate that is freeze-dried and vapor-treated. It has clottable protein (75 to 115 mg), fibrinogen (70 to 110 mg), plasma fibronectin (2 to 9 mg), factor XIII (10 to 50 IU), and plasminogen (40 to 120 micrograms). The small blue bottle contains aprotinin solution, which is bovine derived (3000 KIU/mL). The white bottle has thrombin 4 from bovine source and is freeze-dried (500 IU/mL). The small black bottle contains calcium chloride solution of 40 mmol/L. The vials are warmed for several minutes, and the fibrinolysis inhibitor, aprotinin, is added to the sealer protein concentrate vial followed by warming and stirring. The second component is prepared by injecting the calcium chloride into the vial of thrombin. It is important to use separate syringes and needles for preparation, otherwise premature clotting can occur. The VH form has bovine fibrinolysis inhibitor solution, while the Tisseel kit has synthetic fibrinolysis inhibitor solution.

The adhesive properties are created by combining the 2 components. This can be done by using an injector that has a parallel syringe system; the fibrin sealer solution would be placed in one syringe and the thrombin solution in the other. They are combined in the cone at the end of the 2 syringes and delivered through a common barrel (Duploject system). For ophthalmic uses, because of the small amounts delivered, it may be more convenient to apply the solutions through different syringes onto the tissues, activating the adhesive properties when they make contact with each other and allowing the thrombin to convert the fibrinogen to fibrin. The concentration of the thrombin determines the rate of conversion. The more concentrated the thrombin solution, the faster the clot forms. The clot can form in 10 seconds for the most concentrated solution, and 60 seconds through diluting the solution from 500 IU/mL to 4 IU/mL. A dry field is important for proper adhesion.

Artiss fibrin sealant was approved for topical application for the adherence of autologous skin grafts to surgically prepared wound beds resulting from burns in 2008. It is available as a freeze-dried kit stored between 2°C and 25°C, or as a pre-filled syringe that is frozen at temperatures below -20°C. It is available in 2, 4, and 10 mL pack sizes. After reconstitution, the product should be used within 4 hours. With the typical dilution of this product, the surgeon has approximately 60 seconds to manipulate the tissue prior to polymerization. Final strength is achieved in approximately 2 hours. The amount of fibrinogen in the sealer protein solution is 100 mg/mL, and the synthetic fibrinolysis inhibitor is 3000 KIU/mL. Human albumin is also in this solution. In the thrombin solution, approximately 4 units/mL of human thrombin are present along with 40 umol/mL of calcium chloride. Vapor heating and solvent/detergent treatment processes are used to reduce the chances of viral transmission.

Evicel fibrin sealant was approved in the United States in 2003. It was approved for hemostasis in patients undergoing surgery and is a frozen solution. One vial of the solution contains fibrinogen at a concentration around 70 mg/mL, and the other has thrombin at around 1000 IU/mL. It is stored at temperatures below -18°C, and, once thawed, should be used within 24 hours if kept at room temperature. Evicel contains no bovine protein components.

Risks

Because common fibrin adhesives are prepared from pooled donor sources, there is some risk of infection transmission, although this risk is very low.[9-15] Donors are tested for viral markers and tested again 6 months after donation. Most of the products are also sterilized by gamma irradiation or solvent/detergent treatments.

Anaphylactic reactions following its application have been reported.[16,17] This reaction has been attributed to the presence of aprotinin in fibrin glue.

Ophthalmic Uses

Fibrin sealant has many applications in ophthalmology, partially because it forms a smooth seal along the wound edge, has significant resistance to shearing stress, and reduces bleeding.[18]

As early as 1986, the glue was used in conjunctival surgery utilizing pericardium. Amniotic membrane transplantation in conjunctivochalasis has also been reported with fibrin glue.[19] The major use with conjunctival surgery is in pterygium surgery.[20-26] It is associated with less inflammation than sutures, a shorter surgical time, and less postoperative discomfort. It has also been used for closure of the conjunctiva after other surgical procedures such as strabismus surgery.[27-29]

Fibrin adhesive has also been used in corneal surgery for corneal perforations and melts, or for sealing amniotic membrane over corneal ulcers.[30-32] It has also been used to fixate lamellar grafts[33-36] and for fixating donor limbal lenticules in limbal cell transplantation.[37]

Fibrin adhesive has also been used in refractive surgery to assist in the management of recurrent epithelial ingrowth after laser in-situ keratomileusis (LASIK).[38-41] Mechanical débridement is first performed and fibrin glue is used in the gutter of the LASIK flap to reduce regrowth of epithelium under the flap by providing a slowly dissolving barrier against the growing epithelium. It can be combined with flap suturing if sutures are needed to seal a large fistula.[41] The glue is opaque, and the visual recovery is slower than débridement of the epithelium alone. It has also been used in photorefractive keratectomy to reduce corneal haze.[42]

In glaucoma surgery, conjunctival closure can be performed with fibrin glue.[43] Leaking blebs have also been sealed with fibrin adhesives.[44-46] The glue has been used for temporary closure of scleral flaps after trabeculectomy in eyes with hypotony as well.[44]

Fibrin sealant has also been used to seal cataract surgery incisions.[47-52] The haptics of the IOL can be secured to the sclera with fibrin adhesive.[53] In the area of vitreoretinal surgery, it has been reported to successfully seal full thickness macular holes.[54-56] Conjunctival wound closure after retinal detachment surgery is another reported use.[57,58]

Fibrin glue has also been used for lid and adnexal surgery, such as for repairing lacerated canaliculi and attaching lacrimal and nasal mucosal flaps.[59,60] Other soft tissue and reconstructive uses are possible.[61-63]

Two-part thrombin fibrin adhesives have a long track history of use in surgery. Fibrin adhesive is a very useful tool in the area of ophthalmology. The dual component nature of the glue makes it very flexible for use in conjunctival, corneal, and retinal uses.

References

1. Rousou J, Levitsky S, Gonzalez-Lavin L, et al. Randomized clinical trial of fibrin sealant in patients undergoing resternotomy or reoperation after cardiac operations; a multicenter study. *J Thorac Cardiovasc Surg.* 1989;97:194-203.
2. McCarthy PM, Borsh J, Cosgrove DM. Fibrin sealant: the Cleveland Clinic Experience. In: Schlag G, Wolner E, Eckersberger F, eds. *Fibrin Sealing in Surgical and Non-Surgical Fields, Volume 6: Cardiovascular Surgery, Thoracic Surgery.* Berlin, Germany: Springer-Verlag; 1995.
3. Tidrick RT, Warner ED. Fibrin fixation of skin transplant. *Surgery.* 1944;15:90-95.
4. Katzin HM. Aqueous fibrin fixation of corneal transplants in the rabbit. *Arch Ophthalmol.* 1945;35:415-420.
5. Thompson DF, Letassy NA, Thompson GD. Fibrin glue: a review of its preparation, efficacy, and adverse effects as a topical hemostat. *Drug Intell Clin Pharm.* 1988;22:946-952.
6. Chabbat J, Tellier M, Porte P, Steinbuch M. Properties of a new fibrin glue stable in liquid state. *Thromb Res.* 1994;15:525-533.
7. Le Guéhennec L, Layrolle P, Daculsi G. A review of bioceramics and fibrin sealant. *Eur Cell Mater.* 2004;8:1-10.
8. Forseth M, O'Grady K, Toriumi DM. The current status of cyanoacrylate and fibrin tissue adhesives. *J Long Term Eff Med Implants.* 1992;2:221-233.
9. Siedentop KH, Park JJ, Shah AN, Bhattacharya TK, O'Grady KM. Safety and efficacy of currently available fibrin tissue adhesives. *Am J Otolaryngol.* 2001;22:230-235.
10. Evenson SA, Rollag H. Solvent/detergent-treated clotting factors and hepatitis A virus seroconversion. *Lancet.* 1993;341:971-972.
11. Lefrere JJ, Mariotti M, Thauvin M. B19 parvovirus DNA in solvent/detergent-treated anti-haemophilia concentrates. *Lancet.* 1994;343:211-212.
12. Everts PA, Knape JT, Weibrich G, et al. Platelet-rich plasma and platelet gel: a review. *J Extra Corpor Technol.* 2006;38:174-187.
13. Dohan DM, Choukroun J, Diss A, et al. Platelet-rich fibrin (PRF): a second-generation platelet concentrate. Part I: technological concepts and evolution. *Oral Surg Oral Med Oral Pathol Oral Radiol Endod.* 2006;101:37-44.
14. Aizawa P, Winge S, Karlsson G. Large-scale preparation of thrombin from human plasma. *Thromb Res.* 2008;122:560-567.
15. Alston SM, Solen KA, Sukavaneshvar S, Mohammad SF. In vivo efficacy of a new autologous fibrin sealant. *J Surg Res.* 2008;146:143-148.
16. Shirari T, Shimota H, Chida K, Sano S, Takeuchi Y, Yasueda H. Anaphylaxis to aprotinin in fibrin sealant. *Intern Med.* 2005;44:1088-1089.
17. Beieriein W, Scheule AM, Antoniadis G, Braun C, Schosser R. Anaphylaxis. *Transfusion.* 2000;40:302-305.
18. Berguer R, Staerkel RL, Moore EE, Moore FA, Galloway WB, Mockus MB. Use of fibrin glue in deep hepatic wounds. *J Trauma.* 1991;31:408-411.
19. Kheirkhah A, Casas V, Blanco G, et al. Amniotic membrane transplantation with fibrin glue for conjunctivochalasis. *Am J Ophthalmol.* 2007;144:311-313.

20. Uy HS, Reyes JM, Flores JD, Lim-Bon-Siong R. Comparison of fibrin glue and sutures for attaching conjunctival autografts after pterygium excision. *Ophthalmology.* 2005;112:667-671.

21. Bahar I, Weinberger D, Dan G, Avisar R. Pterygium surgery. *Cornea.* 2006;25:1168-1172.

22. Marticorena J, Rodríguez-Ares MT, Touriño R, et al. Pterygium surgery: conjunctival autograft using a fibrin adhesive. *Cornea.* 2006;25:34-36.

23. Bahar I, Weinberger D, Gaton DD, Avisar R. Fibrin glue versus vicryl sutures for primary conjunctival closure in pterygium surgery: long-term results. *Curr Eye Res.* 2007;32:399-405.

24. Jiang J, Yang Y, Zhang M, Fu X, Bao X, Yao K. Comparison of fibrin sealant and sutures for conjunctival autograft fixation in pterygium surgery: one year follow up. *Ophthalmologica.* 2008;222:105-111.

25. Jain AK, Bansal R, Sukhija J. Human amniotic membrane transplantation with fibrin glue in management of primary pterygia: a new tuck-in technique. *Cornea.* 2008;27:94-99.

26. Kheirkhah A, Gasas V, Sheha H, Raju VK, Tseng SC. Role of conjunctival inflammation in surgical outcome after amniotic membrane transplantation with or without fibrin glue for pterygium. *Cornea.* 2008;27:56-63.

27. Spierer A, Barequet I, Rosner M, Solomon AS, Martinowitz U. Reattachment of extraocular muscles using fibrin glue in a rabbit model. *Invest Ophthalmol Vis Sci.* 1997;38:543-546.

28. Erbil H, Sinav S, Sullu Y, Kandemir B. An experimental study on the use of fibrin sealants in strabismus surgery. *Turk J Pediatr.* 1991;33:111-116.

29. Biedner B, Rosenthal G. Conjunctival closure in strabismus surgery: Vicryl versus fibrin glue. *Ophthalmic Surg Lasers.* 1996;27:967-970.

30. Lagoutte FM, Gauther L, Comte PRM. A fibrin sealant for perforated and preperforated corneal ulcers. *Br J Ophthalmol.* 1989;73:757-761.

31. Vrabec MP, Jordan JJ. A surgical technique for the treatment of central corneal perforations. *J Ref Corneal Surg.* 1994;10:365-367.

32. Hick S, Demers PE, Brunette I, La C, Mabon M, Duchesne B. Amniotic membrane transplantation and fibrin glue in the management of corneal ulcers and perforations: a review of 33 cases. *Cornea.* 2005;24:369-377.

33. Ibrahim-Elzembely HA, Kaufman SC, Kaufman HE. Human fibrin tissue glue for corneal lamellar adhesion in rabbits: a preliminary study. *Cornea.* 2003;22:735-739.

34. Kaufman HE, Insler MS, Ibrahim-Elzembely HA, Kaufman SC. Human fibrin tissue adhesive for sutureless lamellar keratoplasty and scleral patch adhesion: a pilot study. *Ophthalmology.* 2003;110:2168-2172.

35. Duarte MC, Kim T. Sutureless lamellar keratoplasty: a modified approach for fibrin glue application. *Cornea.* 2007;26:1127-1128.

36. Narendran N, Mohamed S, Shah S. No sutures corneal grafting—a novel use of overlay sutures and fibrin glue in Deep Anterior Lamellar Keratoplasty. *Contact Lens Anterior Eye.* 2007;30:207-209.

37. Pfister RR, Sommers CL. Fibrin sealant in corneal stem cell transplantation. *Cornea.* 2005;24:593-598.

38. Anderson NJ, Hardten DR. Fibrin glue for the prevention of epithelial ingrowth after laser in situ keratomileusis. *J Cataract Refract Surg.* 2003;29:1425-1429.

39. Yeh DL, Bushley DM, Kim T. Treatment of traumatic LASIK flap dislocation and epithelial ingrowth with fibrin glue. *Am J Ophthalmol.* 2006;141:960-962.

40. Rapuano CJ. Management of epithelial ingrowth after laser in situ keratomileusis on a tertiary care cornea service. *Cornea.* 2010;29:307-313.

41. Narvaez J, Chakrabarty A, Chang K. Treatment of epithelial ingrowth after LASIK enhancement with a combined technique of mechanical débridement, flap suturing, and fibrin glue application. *Cornea.* 2006;25:1115-1117.

42. Bonatti JA, Bechara SJ, Dall'Col MW, Cresta FB, Carricondo PC, Kara-Jose N. A fibrin-related line of research and theoretical possibilities for the use of fibrin glue as a temporary basal membrane in non-perforated corneal ulcers and in photorefractive keratectomy (PRK)-operated corneas. *Arq Bras Oftalmol.* 2007;70;884-889.

43. O'Sullivan F, Dalton R, Rostron LK. Fibrin glue: an alternative method of wound closure in glaucoma surgery. *J Glaucoma.* 1996;5:367-370.

44. Grewing R, Mester U. Fibrin sealant in the management of complicated hypotony after trabeculectomy. *Ophthalmic Surg Lasers.* 1997;28:124-127.

45. Wright MM, Brown EA, Maxwell K, Cameron JD, Walsh AW. Laser-cured fibrinogen glue to repair bleb leaks in rabbits. *Arch Ophthalmol.* 1998;116:199-202.

46. Seligsohn A, Moster MR, Steinmann W, Fontanarosa J. Use of Tisseel fibrin sealant to manage bleb leaks and hypotony: case series. *J Glaucoma.* 2004;13:227.

47. Mester U, Zuche M, Rauber M. Astigmatism after phacoemulsification with posterior chamber lens implantation: small incision technique with fibrin adhesive for wound closure. *J Cataract Refract Surg.* 1993;19:616-619.

48. Alio JL, Mulet E, Sakla HF, Gobbi F. Efficacy of synthetic and biological bioadhesives in scleral tunnel Phaco in eyes with high myopia. *J Cataract Refract Surg.* 1998;24:983-988.

49. Grewing R, Mester U. Radial suture stabilized by fibrin glue to correct preoperative against-the-rule astigmatism during cataract surgery. *Ophthalmic Surg.* 1994;25:446-448.

50. Mester U. Wound closure with fibrin adhesive in cataract surgery. In: Schlag G, Ascher PW, Steinkogler FJ, Stammberger H, eds. *Fibrin Sealing in Surgical and Non-Surgical Fields, Volume 5: Neurosurgery, Ophthalmic Surgery, ENT.* Berlin, Germany: Springer-Verlag; 1994;123-132.

51. Rauber M, Mester U, Zuche M. Fibrin adhesive for wound closure in small-incision cataract surgery. In: Schlag G, Ascher PW, Steinkogler FJ, Stammberger H, eds. *Fibrin Sealing in Surgical and Non-Surgical Fields, Volume 5: Neurosurgery, Ophthalmic Surgery, ENT.* Berlin, Germany: Springer-Verlag; 1994;116-122.

52. Henrick A, Kalpakian B, Gaster RN, Vanley C. Organic tissue glue in the closure of cataract incisions in rabbit eyes. *J Cataract Refract Surg.* 1991;17:551-555.

53. Agarwal A, Kumar DA, Jacob S, Baid C, Agarwal A, Srinivasan S. Fibrin glue-assisted sutureless posterior chamber intraocular lens implantation in eyes with deficient posterior capsules. *J Cataract Refract Surg.* 2008;34:1433-1438.

54. Tilanus MAD, Deutman T, Deutman AF. Full-thickness macular holes treated with vitrectomy and tissue glue. *Int Ophthalmol.* 1994/1995;18:355-358.

55. Olsen TW, Sternberg P Jr, Capone A Jr, et al. Macular hole surgery using thrombin-activated fibrinogen and selective removal of the internal limiting membrane. *Retina.* 1998;18:322-329.

56. Blumenkranz MS, Ohana E, Shaikh S, et al. Adjuvant methods in macular hole surgery: intraoperative plasma-thrombin mixture and postoperative fluid-gas exchange. *Ophthalmic Surg Lasers.* 2001;32:198-207.

57. Zauberman H, Hemo I. Use of fibrin glue in ocular surgery. *Ophthalmic Surg.* 1988;19:132-133.

58. Mentens R, Stalmans P. Comparison of fibrin glue and sutures for conjunctival closure in pars plana vitrectomy. *Am J Ophthalmol.* 2007;144:128-131.

59. Steinkogler FJ. Fibrin tissue adhesive for the repair of lacerated canaliculi lacrimales. In: Schlag G, Redl H, eds. *Fibrin Sealant in Operative Medicine, Volume 2: Ophthalmology-Neurosurgery.* Berlin, Germany: Springer-Verlag; 1986;92-94.

60. Steinkogler FJ, Moser E. Caniculo-cystostomy using the fibrin glue technique. *Fortschr Ophthalmol.* 1989;86:76-77.

61. Gosain AK, Lyon VB. Plastic Surgery Educational Foundation DATA Committee. The current status of tissue glues: part II. For adhesion of soft tissues. *Plastic Reconstr Surg.* 2002;110:1581-1585.

62. Steinkogler FJ, Kuchar A. Fibrin sealant in ophthalmic plastic and reconstructive surgery. In: Schlag G, Ascher PW, Steinkogler FJ, Stammberger H, eds. *Fibrin Sealing in Surgical and Non-Surgical Fields, Volume 5: Neurosurgery, Ophthalmic Surgery, ENT.* Berlin, Germany: Springer-Verlag; 1994:87-96.

63. Mandel MA. Closure of blepharoplasty incisions with autologous fibrin glue. *Arch Ophthalmol.* 1990;108:842-844.

5

5-Fluorouracil and Mitomycin-C
Adjuncts to Pterygium Surgery

M. Camille Almond, MD; B. Travis Dastrup, MD;
and Stephen C. Kaufman, MD, PhD

Simple excision of a primary pterygium is usually considered a fairly clear-cut procedure. Some ophthalmology training programs allow their first and second year residents to perform pterygium excision among their earliest surgical procedures, viewing this as a straightforward surgery appropriate for the novice surgeon. While many of these lesions can be readily removed to the initial satisfaction of both surgeon and patient, the recurrence rate can be disappointingly high, with reports averaging between 30% and 50% in most studies, but as high as 89% in others.[1,2] Numerous surgical techniques and adjunctive therapies have been proposed and evaluated in an effort to produce more favorable and consistent results.[1-8] Antimetabolites, 5-fluorouracil (5-FU), and mitomycin-C (MMC) have been used to decrease the recurrence rate of pterygia and generate more predictable surgical outcomes.

5-Fluorouracil

Basic Science

5-FU is a fluorinated pyrimidine, first synthesized by Dushinski, Pleven, and Heidelberger in 1957.[9,10] Its primary antimetabolic effect is believed to be inhibition of thymidylate synthetase; this leads to a lack of intracellular thymidine, a component that is necessary for DNA production. Additional effects of 5-FU are attributed to inhibition of other enzymes or the incorporation of its metabolites into RNA.[10,11] Exposure to 5-FU poses a significant impediment to the proliferation of conjunctival and Tenon's capsule fibroblasts and that of corneal epithelial cells.[10-17] Its theoretical effect in preventing the recurrence of pterygia derives from this inhibitory action on fibroblast proliferation.

Hovanesian JA. *Pterygium: Techniques and*
Technologies for Surgical Success (pp 55-64)

TABLE 5-1. STUDIES INVOLVING INTRAOPERATIVE 5-FLUOROURACIL

YEAR	REFERENCE	TYPE OF STUDY	CONTROL	5-FU DOSE	NO. OF EYES	TYPE OF SURGERY	RECURRENCE 5-FU	RECURRENCE CONTROL
2009	Valezi et al[18]	P	None	25 mg/mL*	125	Conjunctival approximation	35.8%	n/a
2008	Bekibele et al[19]	R	Conjunctival autograft	50 mg/mL†	68	Bare sclera with anchoring of conjunctival edges with 8-0 silk	11.4%	12.4%
2004	Bekibele et al[20]	Rtr	Beta-irradiation	25 mg/mL††	55	Bare sclera	25.9%	22.5%
2003	Akarsu et al[21]	P	None	25 mg/mL‡	28	Conjunctival approximation	25%	n/a
1995	Maldonado et al[22]	RM	Distilled water	10 mg/mL‡‡	40	Bare sclera	60%	35%

Study Type:
P = Prospective without control
R = Randomized controlled prospective study (unmasked)
RM = Randomized, double-masked, placebo-controlled study
Rtr = Retrospective nonrandomized review of cases

5-FU Dosing Regimen:
*0.2 mL 5-FU (25 mg/mL) injected subconjunctivally.[18]
†Weck-cel sponge soaked in 5-FU (50 mg/mL) for 5 minutes, wetting the sponge with one drop of 5-FU every minute, then 1 minute of copious irrigation with saline solution.[19]
††Weck-cel sponge soaked in 5-FU (25 mg/mL) for 5 minutes, wetting the sponge with one drop of 5-FU every minute, then 1 minute of copious irrigation with saline solution.[20]
‡Sponge soaked in 5-FU (25 mg/mL) for 3 minutes, then rinsed with balanced salt solution.[21]
‡‡Sponge saturated with 5-FU (10 mg/mL) for 5 minutes, then irrigated with saline solution.[22]

Clinical Experience

The recurrence rate following intraoperative 5-FU injection is rather uninspiring, with rates between 11.4% and 60% (Table 5-1).[18-22] The largest reported series to date included 125 consecutive eyes with intraoperative 5-FU (25 mg/mL) that found a 35.8% recurrence rate.[18] A randomized, though unmasked, trial comparing a higher dose of 5-FU (50 mg/mL) showed a lower recurrence rate (11.4%) but was statistically no better than conjunctival autograft (12.4%). The authors advocate an additional randomized study where the treatment group receives 5-FU and a conjunctival autograft.[19] Ideally, such a study would also be double-masked with the same surgical technique for the 5-FU group as for the control group. Unfortunately, no such study has been performed to date. The existing published data fail to give strong support for routine use of intraoperative 5-FU (see Table 5-1), although there may be a role for postoperative 5-FU, particularly in treating recurrent lesions.[21-24]

Prabhasawat et al published the results of an unmasked, randomized, prospective, controlled clinical trial of 5-FU injection for "impending recurrent pterygium."[4] They used a grading system involving characteristics of the recurrent pterygium, and then enrolled patients with grade 3 lesions. This grade corresponded to the presence of fibrovascular tissue at the surgical site that had not yet extended onto the cornea. These 109 eyes were deemed to be at high risk for a recurrence. Patients were randomized to either a control group of topical steroids or to 1 of 2 treatment groups: two 5 mg (0.1 mL) 5-FU intralesional injections separated by 1 week, or 1 dose of 20 mg of intralesional triamcinolone. The 5-FU group also received hourly irrigation with an artificial tear drop for 3 days in an effort to reduce the risk of corneal complications. The respective recurrence rates were 31.4% in controls, 7.7% with 5-FU, and 14.3% with triamcinolone. The difference between the 5-FU group and the control was statistically significant (P=0.009). Corneal complications were common in the 5-FU group, mostly mild and limited to punctate epithelial erosions, but larger areas involving greater than 30% of the corneal surface were seen in 3 patients. All of the corneal complications noted in this study eventually resolved.[24]

Complications

Although the literature for 5-FU use in pterygia is relatively sparse, only minor and transient complications have been reported in conjunction with its use in this context.[25] However, there are many more published reports of its use in the glaucoma literature, and a number of serious complications have been described. These complications include persistent epithelial defects, spontaneous bleb rupture, and development of a bacterial ulcer leading to perforation. The usual dosage (up to 105 mg in 2 weeks[26]), however, was much higher than has been suggested for use in pterygia, which is a total dose of between 10 and 20 mg for injections.[21,24] Weinreb recommended dosage adjustments to minimize corneal complications after filtration surgery.[27] The total dose ranged between 17.5 to 62.5 mg in his study, with some small overlap with the range advocated in pterygia. Epithelial changes were noted in 29% of patients, including epithelial defects in 16%. Though these resolved with cessation of the 5-FU injections, they do suggest some risk to the cornea. Lee et al reported development of a large epithelial defect that did not heal until 6 weeks after glaucoma surgery.[28] Hickey-Dwyer and Wishart reported a case where only a total of 10-mg dose of 5-FU was given (5 mg during surgery and 5 mg the next day) and a large epithelial defect formed.[27,29] The patient went on to develop a corneal infection with abscess formation. This case demonstrates potential toxicity of 5-FU even at the lower doses advocated for pterygium surgery, and shows that epithelial complications can lead to serious corneal infections. Knapp et al reported 2 patients with bacterial corneal ulcers: one with a sterile corneal perforation and another with a corneal plaque and underlying sterile infiltrate.[30] These all occurred in patients with pre-existing corneal abnormalities and suggests that use of 5-FU is relatively contraindicated in patients with pre-existing compromise to their corneal epithelium. Finally, cicatricial ectropion with topical 5-FU and punctal-canalicular stenosis with systemic 5-FU have been reported.[31,32]

Mitomycin-C

Basic Science

MMC is an antibiotic and antineoplastic agent that was first isolated from the bacterium *Streptomyces caespitosus*. It undergoes reductive activation to become a potent alkylating agent. Under hypoxic conditions, it interferes with DNA replication by cross-linking DNA, usually at the N^2 position of guanine; as such it is most effective in cells that are actively dividing. Under aerobic conditions, it generates toxic oxygen radicals capable of nonspecific interference with RNA and protein synthesis.[33] It has been used intravenously as an antineoplastic agent against tumors of the gastrointestinal tract, pancreas, lung, and breast, among others. It has also been used in an intravascular application for bladder cancer.

Clinical Experience

Based on its toxicity in actively dividing cells, MMC has been proposed as an adjuvant for use in pterygium surgery as an inhibitor of fibroblast activity. Its use in this capacity was first described in 1963 by Kunimoto and Mori in Japan, but was later popularized in Western literature in 1988, when Singh et al described its use in various concentrations for application following pterygium excision.[34,35] This article described masked randomization to placebo versus topical 1.0 mg/mL MMC application every 6 hours following pterygium excision to bare sclera, for a total of 14 days. Given early development of conjunctival and corneal irritation with excessive tearing in the 1.0 mg/mL MMC group, the dosage was decreased to 0.4 mg/mL during the course of the study, such that results were reported for 3 different treatment groups. Recurrence at 6 months was 2.2% for the MMC-treated groups combined and 88.9% for the placebo group; multiple authors have since corroborated the significant reduction in recurrence rates with MMC as an adjunct to surgical excision.[36-45] In this study, there were subjective complaints of tearing, photophobia, and pain in all groups that persisted for a longer period of time in the 1.0 mg/mL MMC group as compared to the other 2 groups, both of which showed resolution of symptoms by week 3. On average, the MMC groups showed delayed conjunctival re-epithelialization by about 2 weeks. Other studies later demonstrated favorable results in regard to recurrence rates and complications with even lower doses of MMC. Hayasaka et al described 0.02% MMC application for 5 days following resection with a decrease in recurrence from 32% to 7% in primary pterygium and from 45% to 9% in recurrent pterygium compared to resection alone at a 3- to 8-year postoperative review.[36] Frucht-Pery and Ilsar reported equivalent outcomes with postoperative 0.01% MMC when compared to each postoperative 0.02% MMC and postoperative beta irradiation, at a mean follow-up period of 15.3 months; there were no reported complications beyond postoperative irritation in the 0.01% group, which was equal in duration (3 weeks) to the other 2 groups.[37]

Although Singh et al later published long-term follow-up results (mean 18 months)[38] on their original series of MMC-treated patients, reiterating its safety and efficacy and a continued lack of recurrence in the MMC group relative to placebo, subsequent published reports have described the development of severe complications, even many months after a seemingly uncomplicated initial postoperative course.[42,46-49] Adverse events following postoperative topical MMC include cataract formation, anterior uveitis, scleral plaque and necrosis, corneal edema and ulceration, and protracted pain, to name a few. In 1992, Rubinfeld et al described a series of 10 patients with severe complications following instillation of MMC 0.2 to 0.4 mg/mL for 6 days to several weeks postoperatively due to variable patient compliance with instructions.[46] Complications included severe pain, anterior chamber inflammation, nonhealing conjunctival, and corneal and scleral defects, all of which occurred within 1 year of treatment. The authors suggest that high cumulative postoperative doses of MMC may have contributed to the development of these problems. They additionally noted potential predisposing conditions present in these patients including acne rosacea, ichthyosis, and dry eye syndrome, which may have made them more susceptible to complications such as delayed or improper healing. It is suggested that careful patient selection is necessary if one is to use this medication at all in conjunction with pterygium surgery. In 2000, Hayasaka et al described a late development of complications in 4 of their patients treated with the 0.4 mg/mL dosing of postoperative MMC drops (18 to 25 years after pterygium excision).[47] All 4 patients presented with discomfort of the operative eye and were noted on exam to have a calcified plaque at the excision site; at the time of surgical removal of the plaques, scleral thinning was discovered in all cases, necessitating scleral patch grafts.

Another approach to adjunctive MMC application is to apply it intraoperatively in a single dose of 0.2 to 0.4 mg/mL (0.02% to 0.04%) directly to bare sclera for a period of 2 to 5 minutes followed by irrigation with copious balanced salt solution (BSS). This allows for a controlled application and eliminates the concern that patients' misuse or overuse of postoperative drops may be a factor in the development of adverse events. Frucht-Pery et al described a decrease in recurrence from 45% to 5% in patients randomized to a 5-minute intraoperative application of 0.02% MMC versus placebo (NaCl 0.9%) using a bare sclera surgical technique, with no complications noted in the MMC group at a mean of 8.9 months follow-up.[45] Cardillo et al performed a masked, prospective, randomized study with patients divided into 5 groups: groups 1 and 2 received intraoperative application of 0.02% or 0.04% MMC for 3 minutes, respectively, and groups 3 and 4 received postoperative 0.02% MMC drops 3 times daily for 7 days or 0.04% MMC 3 times daily for 14 days, respectively.[40] The fifth group was a control group with surgical excision alone and no adjuvant used. The authors demonstrated equal reduction in recurrence across all treatment groups (between 4% and 6.6% recurrence at 28-month follow-up) from a control rate of 29.27%, with complications limited to mild superficial keratitis, which was self-limited and occurred equally in all groups, including controls. They therefore recommend using the lowest intraoperative dose (0.02%) given similar efficacy with greater surgeon control of time and concentration of application, and potentially less long-term effects secondary to medication toxicity. It should be noted that postoperative drops were provided in a very controlled fashion (only the exact volume recommended for the postoperative course) and that the surgical technique included rotation of a conjunctival flap over the excision site at the conclusion of each case. It is quite possible that these procedural modifications contributed to the lack of severe complications in this study; in a 1993 comment in *Ophthalmology,* Penna suggested the potent avascular effect of MMC may have precipitated later corneal and scleral ulceration in eyes treated with adjuvant MMC following the bare sclera excision technique.[50] Rotation of a conjunctival graft over the defect following MMC application may lessen this risk by providing a functional vascular supply. Unfortunately, even with these modifications, there have been serious adverse events reported. Dougherty et al described a case of severe corneoscleral melt necessitating lamellar graft placement in a patient who had received a 3-minute application of 0.02% MMC followed by a sliding conjunctival flap closure.[51] Figure 5-1 demonstrates a typical scleral melt associated with the intraoperative use of MMC.

Conclusion

It is clear from the review of existing literature that considerable debate still exists as to the safest and most effective use of antimetabolite adjuncts in the setting of pterygium surgery.[52-57] The published series to date give little support for advocating routine use of intraoperative 5-FU. A study of 5-FU versus placebo with conjunctival autograft may be helpful in the future. Postoperative 5-FU in impending recurrent

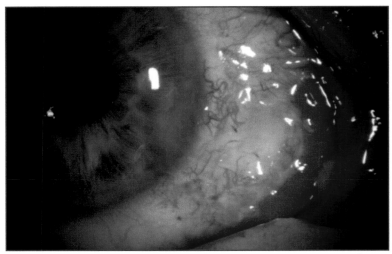

Figure 5-1. A scleral melt, in progress, after using intraoperative MMC during surgery for a recurrent pterygium. Note the white, avascular scleral melt and its affected surrounding area. The melt eventually stabilized and healed with lubrication, a prophylactic topical antibiotic, and close observation.

pterygium shows promise, but without more clinical experience, caution must be exercised in applying its use as a surgical adjuvant. Safety must be monitored over the long term, and it likely should be avoided in patients with corneal epithelial disease.

Recent publications indicate that many surgeons continue to utilize MMC in the treatment of primary pterygium.[43,44,58] It has been considered an attractive option given low cost, ease of use, shorter surgical times relative to conjunctival autograft or rotational flap, and avoidance of the need for tissue compared to amniotic membrane application. Numerous comparative studies have indicated MMC is at least as efficacious as conjunctival autograft in preventing recurrence.[38,39,59,60] However, Young et al in 2004 showed a possible benefit to limbal conjunctival autograft (LCAU) over MMC,[61] and Cheng et al demonstrated improved outcomes using LCAU in recurrent pterygia relative to MMC (outcomes were similar in the 2 groups for primary pterygium).[58] In fact, Ma et al reported equal reduction in recurrence by simply using amniotic membrane graft compared to postoperative MMC drops.[59]

Currently, 5-FU is not frequently utilized in the setting of pterygium excision, as reflected by the paucity of clinical reports as to its optimal use. With regard to MMC complications, it is advisable to carefully select patients with a low risk for deficient healing, excluding those with conditions such as meibomitis, blepharitis, rosacea, Sjögren's syndrome, and keratoconjunctivitis sicca, and possibly to reserve this medication for intraoperative use in a low concentration only for patients with severe, recurrent pterygia. Neither MMC nor 5-FU is FDA approved for ophthalmic use in the United States; therefore, their use is permissible but considered off-label. The risks, benefits, and potential complications associated with these medications must be discussed with the patient. We look forward to additional studies, new surgical techniques, and newer compounds that may help decrease the recurrence rate of pterygia in a safe and predictable manner.

Supported in part by a grant from Research to Prevent Blindness.

References

1. Hirst LW. The treatment of pterygium. *Surv of Ophthalmol.* 2003;48:145-180.
2. Fernandes M, Sangwan VS, Bansal AK, et al. Outcome of pterygium surgery: analysis over 14 years. *Eye.* 2005;19:1182-1190.
3. Frucht-Pery J, Siganos CS, Ilsar M. Intraoperative application of topical mitomycin C for pterygium surgery. *Ophthalmology.* 1996;103:674-677.
4. Prabhasawat P, Barton K, Burkett G, Tseng SC. Comparison of conjunctival autografts, amniotic membrane grafts, and primary closure for pterygium excision. *Ophthalmology.* 1997;104:974-985.
5. Ma DH, See LC, Liau SB, Tsai RJ. Amniotic membrane graft for primary pterygium: comparison with conjunctival autograft and topical mitomycin C treatment. *Br J Ophthalmol.* 2000;84:973-978.
6. Luanratanakorn P, Ratanapakorn T, Suwan-apichon O, Chuck RS. Randomized controlled study of conjunctival autograft versus amniotic membrane graft in pterygium excision. *Br J Ophthalmol.* 2006;90:1476-1480.
7. Frucht-Pery J, Raiskup F, Ilsar M, et al. Conjunctival autografting combined with low-dose mitomycin C for prevention of primary pterygium recurrence. *Am J Ophthalmol.* 2006;141:1044-1050.
8. Hirst LW. Prospective study of primary pterygium surgery using pterygium extended removal followed by extended conjunctival transplantation. *Ophthalmology.* 2008;115(10):1663-1672.
9. Dushinski R, Pleven E, Heidelberger C. The synthesis of 5-fluoropyrimidines. *J Am Chem Soc.* 1957;79:4559-4560.
10. Smith S, D'Amore PA, Dreyer EB. Comparative toxicity of mitomycin C and 5-fluorouracil in vitro. *Am J Ophthalmol.* 1994;118:332-337.
11. Blumenkranz MS, Hartzer MK, Hajek AS. Selection of therapeutic agents for intraocular proliferative disease: differing antiproliferative activity of the fluoropyrimidines. *Arch Ophthalmol.* 1987;105:396-399.
12. Khaw PT, Sherwood MB, MacKay SL, et al. Five-minute treatments with fluorouracil, floxuridine, and mitomycin have long-term effects on human Tenon's capsule fibroblasts. *Arch Ophthalmol.* 1992;110:1150-1154.
13. Mallick KS, Hajek AS, Parrish RK. Fluorouracil (5-FU) and cytarabine (Ara-C) inhibition of corneal epithelial cell and conjunctival fibroblast proliferation. *Arch Ophthalmol.* 1985;103:1398-1402.
14. Friend J, Shapiro MS, Thoft RA, et al. Hypomitosis of ocular surface epithelium and persistent epithelial defect with 5-fluorouracil. *Invest Ophthalmol Vis Sci.* 1984;25(suppl):77.
15. Viveiros MM, Schellini SA, Candeias J, Padovani CR. Exposicao de fibroblastos da capsula de Tenon normal de portadores de pterigio ao 5-fluorouracil e a mitomicina C [Exposure of normal Tenon's capsule fibroblasts from pterygium to 5-fluorouracil and mitomycin C]. *Arq Bras Oftalmol.* 2007;70(1):73-77.
16. Blumenkranz MS, Ophir A, Claflin AJ, Hajek A. Fluorouracil for the treatment of massive periretinal proliferation. *Am J Ophthalmol.* 1982;94:458-467.
17. Yamamoto T, Varani J, Soong HK, Lichter PR. Effects of 5-fluorouracil and mitomycin C on cultured rabbit subconjunctival fibroblasts. *Ophthalmology.* 1990;97:1204-1210.
18. Valezi VG, Schellini SA, Viveiros MM, Padovani CR. Seguranca e efetividade no tratamento do pterigio usando infiltracao de 5-fluoruracila no intraoperatorio [Safety and efficacy of intraoperative 5-fluorouracil infiltration in pterygium treatment]. *Arq Bras Oftalmolog.* 2009;72(2):169-173.
19. Bekibele CO, Baiyeroju AM, Olusanya BA, et al. Pterygium treatment using 5-FU as adjuvant treatment compared to conjunctiva autograft. *Eye.* 2008;22:31-34.
20. Bekibele CO, Maiyeroju AM, Ajayi BG. 5-fluorouracil vs. beta-irradiation in the prevention of pterygium recurrence. *Int J Clin Pract.* 2004;58(10):920-923.
21. Akarsu C, Taner P, Ergin A. 5-Fluorouracil as chemoadjuvant for primary pterygium surgery: preliminary report. *Cornea.* 2003;22(6):522-526.
22. Maldonado MJ, Cano-Parra J, Navea-Tejerina A, et al. Inefficacy of low-dose intraoperative fluorouracil in the treatment of primary pterygium. *Arch Ophthalmol.* 1995;113:1356-1357.
23. Pikkel J, Porges Y, Ophir A. Halting pterygium recurrence by postoperative 5-fluorouracil. *Cornea.* 2001;20(2):168-171.
24. Prabhasawat P, Tesavibul N, Leelapatranura K, Phonjan T. Efficacy of subconjunctival 5-fluorouracil and triamcinolone injection in impending recurrent pterygium. *Ophthalmology.* 2006;113:1102-1109.
25. Khaw PT, Grierson I, Hitchings RA, Rice NS. 5-Fluorouracil and beyond. *Br J Ophthalmol.* 1991;75:577-578.
26. The Fluorouracil Filtering Study Group. Fluorouracil filtering surgery study one-year follow up. *Am J Ophthalmol.* 1989;108:625-635.

27. Weinreb RN. Adjusting the dose of 5-fluorouracil after filtration surgery to minimize side effects. *Ophthalmology.* 1987;94:564-570.

28. Lee DA, Hersh P, Kersten D, Melamed S. Complications of subconjunctival 5-fluorouracil following glaucoma filtering surgery. *Ophthalmol Surg.* 1987;18(3):187-190.

29. Hickey-Dwyer M, Wishart PK. Serious corneal complication of 5-fluorouracil. *Br J Ophthalmol.* 1993;77:250-251.

30. Knapp A, Heuer DK, Stern GA, Driebe WT. Serious corneal complications of glaucoma filtering surgery with postoperative 5-fluorouracil. *Am J Ophthalmol.* 1987;103:183-187.

31. Galentine P, Sloas H, Hargett N, Cupples HP. Bilateral cicatricial ectropion following topical administration of 5-fluorouracil. *Ann Ophthalmol.* 1981;13(5):575-577.

32. Caravella LP, Burns JA, Zangmeister M. Punctal-canalicular stenosis related to systemic fluorouracil therapy. *Arch Ophthalmol.* 1981;99:284-286.

33. Verweij J, Pineda HM. Mitomycin C: mechanism of action, usefulness and limitations. *Anticancer Drugs.* 1990;1:5-13.

34. Kunitomo N, Mori S. Studies on pterygium. Report IV. A treatment of the pterygium by mitomycin C installation. *Acta Soc Ophthalmol Jpn.* 1963;67:601-607.

35. Singh G, Wilson MR, Foster CS. Mitomycin eye drops as treatment for pterygium. *Ophthalmology.* 1998;95:813-821.

36. Hayasaka S, Noda S, Yamamoto Y, Setogawa T. Postoperative instillation of low-dose mitomycin C in the treatment of primary pterygium. *Am J Ophthalmol.* 1988;106(6):715-718.

37. Frucht-Pery J, Ilsar M. The use of low-dose mitomycin C for prevention of recurrent pterygium. *Ophthalmology.* 1994;101:759-762.

38. Singh G, Wilson MR, Foster CS. Long term follow up study of mitomycin eye drops as adjunctive treatment for pterygia and its comparison with conjunctival autograft transplantation. *Cornea.* 1990;9:331-334.

39. Alpay A, Ugurbas SH, Erdogan B. Comparing techniques for pterygium surgery. *Clin Ophthalmol.* 2009;3:69-74.

40. Cardillo JA, Alves MR, Ambrosio LE, Poterio MB, Jose NK. Single intraoperative application versus postoperative mitomycin C eye drops in pterygium surgery. *Ophthalmology.* 1995;102(12):1949-1952.

41. Hayasaka S, Noda S, Yamamoto Y, Setogawa T. Postoperative instillation of mitomycin C in the treatment of recurrent pterygium. *Ophthalmic Surgery.* 1989;20(8):580-583.

42. Mikaniki E, Rasolinejad SA. Simple excision alone versus simple excision plus mitomycin C in the treatment of pterygium. *Ann Saudi Med.* 2007;27(3):158-160.

43. Raiskup F, Solomon A, Landau D, Ilsar M, Frucht-Pery J. Mitomycin C for pterygium: long term evaluation. *Br J Ophthalmol.* 2004;88(11):1425-1428.

44. Wood TO, Williams EE, Hamilton DL, Williams BL. Pterygium surgery with mitomycin and tarsorrhaphy. *Trans Am Ophthalmol Soc.* 2005;103:108-115.

45. Frucht-Pery J, Ilsar M, Hemo I. Single dosage of mitomycin C for prevention of recurrent pterygium: preliminary report. *Cornea.* 1994;13(5):411-413.

46. Rubinfeld RS, Pfister RR, Stein RM, et al. Serious complications of topical mitomycin-C after pterygium surgery. *Ophthalmology.* 1992;99(11):1647-1654.

47. Hayasaka S, Iwasa Y, Nagaki Y, Kadoi C, Matsumoto M, Hayasaka Y. Late complications after pterygium excision with high dose mitomycin C instillation. *Br J Ophthalmol.* 2000;84(9):1081-1082.

48. Fujitani A, Hayasaka S, Shibuya Y, Noda S. Corneoscleral ulceration and corneal perforation after pterygium excision and topical mitomycin C therapy. *Ophthalmologica.* 1993;207(3):162-164.

49. Ewing-Chow DA, Romanchuk KG, Gilmour GR, Underhill JH, Climenhaga DB. Corneal melting after pterygium removal followed by topical mitomycin C therapy. *Can J Ophthalmol.* 1992;27(4):197-199.

50. Penna EP. Mitomycin-C after pterygium excision [letter]. *Ophthalmology.* 1993;100:976.

51. Dougherty PJ, Hardten DR, Lindstrom RL. Corneoscleral melt after pterygium surgery using a single intraoperative application of mitomycin C. *Cornea.* 1996;15(5):537-540.

52. Todani A, Melki SA. Pterygium: current concepts in pathogenesis and treatment. *Int Ophthalmol Clin.* 2009;49:21-30.

53. Hardten DR, Samuelson TW. Ocular toxicity of mitomycin C. *Int Ophthalmol Clin.* 1999;39:79-90.

54. Singh G. Postoperative instillation of low-dose mitomycin C in the treatment of primary pterygium [letter]. *Am J Ophthalmol.* 1989;107:570-571.

55. Sugar A. Who should receive mitomycin C after pterygium surgery? [editorial]. *Ophthalmology.* 1992;99(11)1645-1646.

56. Singh G. Mitomycin C after pterygium excision [letter]. *Ophthalmology.* 1993;100:976-977.

57. Sugar A. Mitomycin C after pterygium excision [reply]. *Ophthalmology.* 1993;100:997.

58. Cheng HC, Tseng SH, Kao PL, Chen FK. Low-dose intraoperative mitomycin C as chemoadjuvant for pterygium surgery. *Cornea.* 2001;20(1):24-29.

59. Ma DH, See LC, Liau SB, Tsai RJ. Amniotic membrane graft for primary pterygium: comparison with conjunctival autograft and topical mitomycin C treatment. *Br J Ophthalmol.* 2000;84(9):973-978.
60. Mahar PS. Conjunctival autograft versus topical mitomycin C in treatment of pterygium. *Eye.* 1997;11:790-792.
61. Young AL, Leung GY, Wong AK, Cheng LL, Lam DS. A randomized trial comparing 0.02% mitomycin C and limbal conjunctival autograft after excision of primary pterygium. *Br J Ophthalmol.* 2004;88(8):995-997.

6

History of
Amniotic Membranes in
Pterygium Surgery

Juan F. Batlle, MD

The placental membranes were first used in ophthalmology by Roth and Sorsby for the reconstruction of ocular surface anomalies.[1,2] Its primary application in the early part of the 20th century was for the management of chemical burns of the eye.[2] The original dried amniotic tissue was called *amnioplastin*. These original amniotic membranes were grafted fresh without any form of preservation and the results were not very encouraging. The early investigations of these European authors were discontinued until the latter part of the same century when it was introduced into the Soviet Union and Latin America.[3]

Amniotic membranes have multiple salutatory capabilities in the surgical reconstruction of the limbus after surgical removal of the pterygium. The nerve endings exposed by surgery are covered, thus reducing the postoperative pain.[4] There is diminished production of prostaglandin, cytokines, and leukotrienes after application of the amniotic membrane, which explains the reduced inflammatory response.[5] The basal lamina and stromal architecture of the amniotic membrane resembles that of human conjunctiva, specifically the presence of collagen type IV and laminin (Figures 6-1 and 6-2).[6]

This similarity to human conjunctiva makes it ideal for use in human conjunctival replacement. The impermeable nature of the amniotic basal lamina prevents evaporation and loss of electrolytes from the scleral bed. In addition, the basal lamina serves as a platform for the growth of healthy conjunctival and corneal epithelial cells. Finally, there is a barrier effect from the amniotic membrane as the abnormal conjunctival fibroblast is withdrawn physically from the surgical limbus, thus impeding recurrence.[7] Kim and Tseng refer to this barrier effect as a substrate that allows restoration of the normal limbal stem cells while precluding the invasion by the abnormal conjunctival stem cells.[8]

The conventional preparation of amniotic tissues described in the literature used glycerol, tissue culture media, and freezing temperatures that required special apparatus for transport. These membranes could not be utilized beyond 3 weeks after preparation. Amniotic membranes prepared originally in the University of Ufa by Professor Muldachev were preserved in 95% ethyl alcohol.[9] The original samples of amniotic membrane were brought to the western hemisphere by Dr. Horacio Serrano

Hovanesian JA. *Pterygium: Techniques and Technologies for Surgical Success (pp 65-78)*

Figure 6-1. The basal lamina of the amniotic membrane.

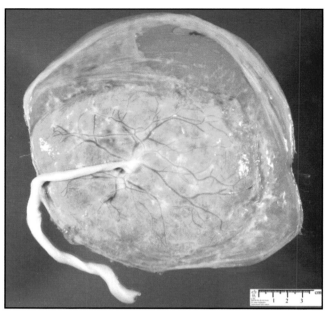

Figure 6-2. Stromal architecture of the amniotic membrane.

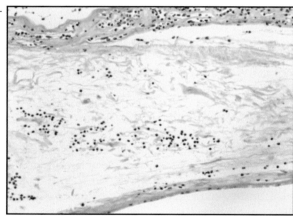

of Venezuela in 1989 (personal communication, March 1991; Figure 6-3). Dr. Serrano was part of a group of Venezuelan ophthalmologists that visited Professor Fyodorov in Moscow to learn the then-popular technique for radial keratotomy. Dr. Serrano was more interested in the use of allotransplants in oculoplastic procedures and was invited to visit the laboratory facilities of Professor Muldachev at the University of Ufa. He visited Ufa and was shown a number of allotransplants for multiple uses in ocular surgery, including orbital prosthesis, tarsal substitutes, scleral substitutes, and the unique substitute for conjunctiva that was labeled *allotransplantat for conjunctiviplasty.* The conjunctival substitute was used routinely in pterygium surgery and Professor Muldachev mentioned its healing properties in the patients that received these membranes after excision of the pterygium. Professor Muldachev described less inflammatory response, less redness and edema, reduced incidence of recurrence, less pain, and faster recovery of the patients that were operated with this particular allotransplant, but he would not identify the origin of the tissue and it remained a secret for several years.[10]

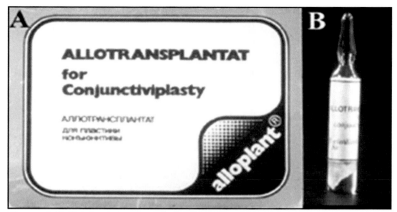

Figure 6-3. Original simples of allotransplantats produced by Muldachev in the late 1980s, were brought to America by Dr. Horacio Serrano of Venezuela. The source of the tissue was not known.

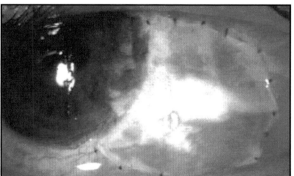

Figure 6-4. First amniotic membrane graft performed with allotransplantats obtained from Professor Muldachev in 1992.

The identification of these samples as true amniotic membrane was accomplished by Dr. Juan Batlle and Dr. Francisco Perdomo of Santo Domingo in 1992, and published as Poster #25 in the American Academy of Ophthalmology Meeting held in Chicago that year.[10] In their original investigation, the histological characteristic of the Soviet membrane provided by Muldachev was described and compared to the membranes obtained from human placenta. The placental membranes were then divided into the chorionic and amniotic layers and the amniotic component was found to be identical to the "mystery tissue" used by Muldachev.[11] This discovery was then presented at the Resident's Day Meeting held by the Bascom Palmer Eye Institute at Key Biscayne in 1992 (Figure 6-4).[12] The membrane had already been utilized in 23 patients with recurrent pterygia, bullous keratopathy, corneal ulcers, dermoid reconstruction and reconstruction of symblepharon, and for corneal dellen. The initial results of this pilot study were comparable to those obtained by Serrano and Muldachev, and the authors encouraged further investigation on this new tissue. Dr. Scheffer Tseng was in the ocular surface department of the Bascom Palmer Eye Institute at the time, and he continued the investigation of this new tissue to confirm the findings of the previous authors. His research led to the creation of the BioTissue laboratory that produces the frozen version of the tissue (Table 6-1).[13]

The process for preservation of amniotic membranes by the BioTissue Company involves a careful removal and separation of the amniotic from the chorionic membrane

TABLE 6-1. HISTORY OF ALLOTRANSPLANTS IN OPHTHALMOLOGY

- Skin—1893
- Oral mucous membrane—1912
- Vaginal mucous membrane—1922
- Tarsal conjunctiva—1938
- Fetal membrane, amnion, and chorion—1948
- Rabbit peritoneum—1941
- Amnion only—1946
- Muldachev's allotransplantat—1980 to 1990

- Serrano brings allotransplantats to Venezuela—1989
- Batlle and Perdomo identify amniotic source of allotransplantat—1992
- Tseng's frozen amniotic membrane (BioTissue)—1993
- Amnion with cultured autologous limbal epithelial cells—2000
- IOP's dry irradiated amniotic membrane (AmbioDry)—2003
- Introduction of tissue glue with amniotic membranes—2004

as described extensively in the literature. The washed membranes are then preserved in a solution of glycerol and TCM in a 50% solution prior to freezing at -80°C. The tissue is transported into the operating room in this deep freeze state and then warmed to room temperature and rehydrated prior to use in the surgical intervention.[13]

In 2003, IOP Ophthalmics (Costa Mesa, CA) developed a new method for the dehydration and mechanical elimination of epithelial cells from human amniotic membranes (Figures 6-5 and 6-6). This product is labeled AmbioDry and it does not require refrigeration or special devices for transportation. It is preserved inside a sterile envelope with a shelf life of 2 years and a convenient design for storage. AmbioDry is prepared by a standard process that carefully excludes contaminated tissue by serologic testing of the donors. The tissue is then cleaned and disinfected. Tissue preservation is achieved by dehydration. The membrane is not subjected to temperatures that could damage the collagen matrix. A unique drying fixture is then employed to emboss texture (design, letters, numbers, or a combination) onto the final graft that will allow identification of stromal and basement membrane sides. Each tissue is then cut to specific sizes and double packaged in disposable foil pouches. The grafts are then terminally sterilized by electron beam sterilization.[14] It is not a freeze-dry process as commonly thought, but the end result is a dry paper-thin membrane that facilitates cutting to adapt to the dimensions of the recipient bed. Once this membrane is moistened with balanced salt solution (BSS) or human tears, it behaves like the naturally occurring conjunctival membrane. The AmbioDry membranes are presented in several thicknesses that are used in different surgical settings. The original AmbioDry is only 40 μm thick, but the AmbioDry 5 measures 120 μm in thickness.

Anatomy and Histology

The human placenta is composed of 2 layers intimately connected by loose connective tissue (Figure 6-7). They are known as the amniotic and chorionic layers. The amniotic layer is the most internal of the 2 layers and comes into contact with the amniotic fluid that surrounds the fetus. Together they form the amniotic sac. The amniotic layer is avascular and lined by simple columnar epithelium overlying a basal membrane that measures 30 to 60 μm in thickness. The chorionic membrane is the outer layer of the sac. It has a stratified columnar epithelium and it is heavily vascularized. The vascular tree originates in the placenta and its ramifications extend to the placental membranes through this chorionic layer. The chorionic layer is separated from the amniotic layer by loose connective tissue and combined; the 2 layers measure 120 to 180 μm.[15]

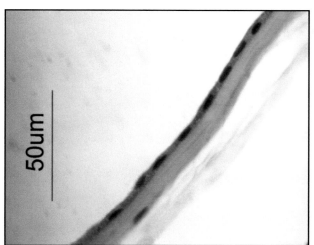

Figure 6-5. Dry human amniotic membrane as processed by IOP Ophthalmics (Costa Mesa, CA).

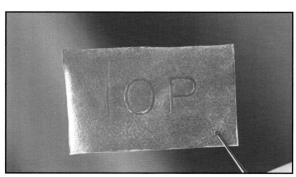

Figure 6-6. AmbioDry histopathological section and appearance of dry human amniotic membrane as processed by IOP Ophthalmics. (Reprinted with permission from IOP Ophthalmics, Inc, Costa Mesa, CA, www.iopinc. com.)

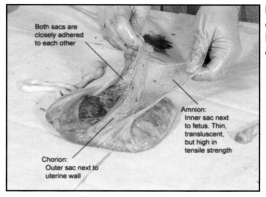

Figure 6-7. The chorionic membrane layer is vascularized and thicker than the amniotic membrane layer, which is shinier and thinner. The 2 layers are easily separated by hand.

The placental membranes have a collagen matrix that is heavily laden with mucopolysaccharides and serve primarily as a protective sac for the developing fetus. The membranes also maintain a barrier for infectious and immunologic agents present in the maternal circulation. Placental membranes have both active and passive transports. Most small molecules and proteins can travel freely through them, but large proteins such as IgM cannot cross through the basal layer. Preservation of the placental membranes in either 95% ethyl alcohol or glycerol mixed in 50-50 proportions with tissue culture media has been utilized for preservation of the amniotic membrane prior

Figure 6-8. Amniotic and chorionic layers. India ink was used to identify the shiny surface that corresponds to the amniotic side of the placental membranes.

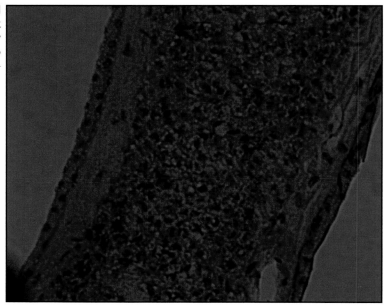

to freezing. These preservatives eliminate the vitality of the placental tissues, thereby making the nuclei pyknotic while the collagen matrix and basal membranes are preserved. Interestingly, both forms of preservation also eliminate the antigenicity of the transplanted membranes and also any potentially virulent agents.[16,17] Preservation is usually accomplished after the amniotic membranes are carefully separated from the chorion (Figures 6-8 and 6-9). The side of the amniotic membrane with the basal lamina and epithelium is shiny and the opposite side facing the chorion is dull. It is important to recognize the difference because the main purpose of the amniotic membrane graft is to provide a substrate covered with a basal membrane that will allow sliding of the new healthy epithelial cells on its surface.[13]

In an outstanding review of the literature, Dua et al[9] described the molecular basis for the functional properties of the amniotic membrane as a tissue substitute.

Cytoskeleton

The cytoskeleton of amniotic membrane cells contains actin, spectrin, erin, cytokeratins, vimentin, and desmoplakin.[18,19] These intracellular filaments participate in the structural integrity of the membrane and also its junctional permeability.[20] Enzymes involved in prostaglandin synthesis such as phospholipases, prostaglandin synthase, and cyclooxygenase have been found in amnion.[5]

Cytokines

Interleukins (IL) 6 and 8 have also been found in association with amniotic cells. ILs are chemotactic agents that attract white blood cells, and both IL-6 and IL-8 are found in high concentrations in the amniotic fluid at birth.[21] IL-1β and IL-1α are receptor antagonists that participate in the regulation of prostaglandin production.[22] Prostaglandin-dehydrogenase, a prostaglandin-inactivating enzyme, was also demonstrated by Cheung et al in the amniotic fluid.[5] IL-4 is also involved in the suppression of activity of prostaglandin-H synthase-2 in amniotic epithelial cells.[5] A number

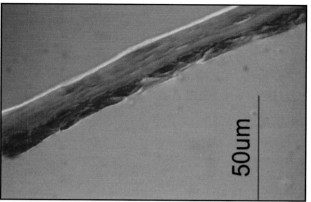

Figure 6-9. Single amniotic membrane layer.

of growth factors were found in human amniotic membrane preserved at -80°C for 1 month. These include epidermal growth factor (EGF,) transforming growth factor alpha (TGF-α), keratinocyte growth factor (KGF), hepatocyte growth factor (HGF), basic fibroblast growth factor (βFGF), TGF, TGF-β1, and TGFβ-3.[23] These studies utilized the polymerase chain reaction for the identification of the messenger ribonucleic acid (mRNA) and also the Enzyme-Linked Immunosorbent Assay (ELISA) test for the protein products. The same investigators found that there was a higher level of these growth factors when the epithelium was preserved than when the epithelium was removed.

Tissue growth factors are also present in significant levels in the amniotic membranes.[24] These include TGF-β1, -β2, and -β3, which, when accompanied by the type I and II receptors, confirm the hypothesis that these growth factors play an important role in regulating the growth of the epithelial cells on the surface of these membranes. EGF receptors have also been found on the amniotic tissues to support this hypothesis.[25]

Endothelin-1 and leukotrienes have been found in amniotic epithelial cells.[6] Carbonic anhydrase isoenzymes are also present and believed to play an important role in the regulation of the amniotic fluid pH.[26] Another component is the secretory leukocyte protease inhibitor, which is a potent inhibitor of leukocyte elastase.[9] These protease inhibitors can be potentiated by IL-1α, IL-1β, and TNF-α, which are believed to play a significant role in the immune-mediated defense mechanism during pregnancy.[6]

The question remains as to how all of these cytokines and immune-mediated proteins are able to survive the denaturation process generated by 95% ethyl alcohol, the irradiation for sterilization, or the effects of glycerol at -80°C and still provide the properties that are attributable by the investigators.[27]

The Matrix

The amniotic membrane matrix is rich in proteoglycans and heparin sulfate. The proteoglycans are particularly important because they are thought to provide the impermeable properties of human amniotic membrane. Collagen I, III, IV, V, and VII; fibronectin; and laminin are also present in the human amnion.[20] Fukuda et al[18] demonstrated that there are similarities between these components both in cornea and conjunctiva. However, he showed that the alpha chain of collagen type IV was similar between human conjunctiva and amnion but different between amniotic membrane and cornea.

Figure 6-10. A pterygium causing severe visual impairment that shows the loss of polarity of the conjunctival epithelial cells and the aggressive invasion of the central cornea by a vascularized pannus.

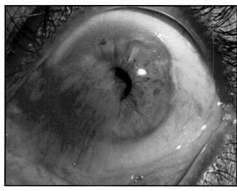

There is evidence that the hemidesmosome integrin α6β4 exhibits a distinct basal location in amniotic epithelium. The basally located integrins promote cell basement membrane attachment and the basolaterally located integrins may be involved in cell-matrix interactions.[19] The basolateral integrins are primarily of the β-1 type and not the α6β4. These components of the matrix act as the "glue" or adherence substrate for the epithelial cells on the surface of the amniotic membrane.

Histopathology

Histopathological studies of pterygia reveal an elastotic degeneration of the conjunctival fibroblasts in the loose connective tissue underlying the body of the pterygium (Figure 6-10). There is also a loss of limbal architecture so that the abnormal conjunctival epithelial cells migrate across the limbus onto the corneal apex. The migration of this fibrovascular pannus originates in the conjunctival tissue, but the pannus then invades the corneal tissue. This maintains a dissection plane just below the level of Bowman's membrane. The fibrovascular traction can involve the plica semilunaris, caruncle, or medial rectus, and in some extreme cases it can produce symblepharon and occlusion of the puncti. This loss of polarity is likely due to loss of normal stem cells in this region as described by Kenyon and Tseng in 1989.[28] This pathologic conversion of epithelial cells and stromal fibroblasts is not fully understood, but there are several theories as to the migratory behavior of these cells.

The most accepted theory in the international ophthalmic literature is that there are environmental factors, such as ultraviolet light exposure of the ocular surface, that cause metaplasia of the conjunctival epithelium and stroma. This theory is supported by epidemiologic studies that have established a correlation between exposure to sunlight and a higher incidence of pterygia as shown by McCarty et al in the region of Victoria, Australia.[29] Lindberg et al[30] published a study that caused a paradigm shift in ophthalmological thinking when they were able to demonstrate very elegantly that corneal stem cells are concentrated in the limbus and that these cells can divide and move in a centripetal fashion, especially when stimulated by trauma. However, this study also showed that central corneal cells do not have this ability, and when injured, are not able to divide (Figure 6-11).

Histological and Physiologic Properties of the Amniotic Membrane

Formation of the amniotic membrane begins after the first week of gestation. It begins as a separation of the inner mass of cells in the germ disk where a slit-like cavity forms a band and expands to become the amniotic cavity. This cavity enlarges by

A Superior Limbus (g) (24%)

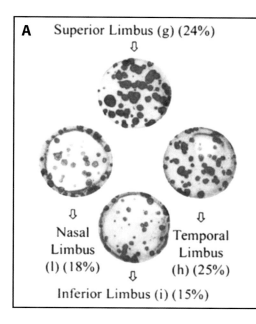

Nasal Limbus (l) (18%) Temporal Limbus (h) (25%)

Inferior Limbus (i) (15%)

B

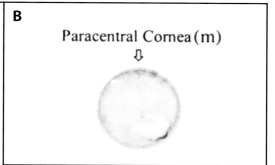

Paracentral Cornea (m)

Figure 6-11. In this study, Dr. Kenyon demonstrated that stem cells (in red) obtained from the paracentral cornea were not able to divide, whereas the limbal stem cells had a great capacity for cell division.

the mitotic division of the amniotic epithelial cells. At the 12th week of gestation, this amniotic sac fuses with the chorionic sac and membranes.[31] The amniotic membrane is truly derived from the mesoderm and mesenchymal tissue of mesodermal origin layers in close apposition to the amniotic membrane to create a thin layer of loose connective tissue, which accounts for the easy separation of the chorion from the amnion.[32]

The amniotic membrane is avascular and its thickness varies between 20 and 60 μm. The 5 layers of the amniotic membrane have been described by Bourne[33] as the following: 1—the epithelial layer, 2—the basement membrane, 3—the compact layer, 4—the fibroblast layer, and 5—the spongy layer. At term, the amnion consists of a thin membrane covered with a simple cuboidal and occasionally columnar epithelium. By light microscopy, the single layer of epithelial cells overlies the basement membrane, which has been studied extensively by scanning electron microscopy. The amniotic basement membrane has tight junctions and its surface is covered with partly amorphous and partly microfibrillar structures with micro processes that firmly adhere this membrane to the epithelial cells. Below the basement membrane is a layer of thin connective tissue composed primarily of collagen, although in some areas of the amniotic membrane, mucin may predominate.[32]

It is this fine ultrastructure that mimics the surface of the normal conjunctival tissues that allows for the salutatory properties of the amniotic membrane when used as a substitute for conjunctival tissues.[34] The normal epithelial cells of the host that receive the amniotic membrane transplant can slide over this familiar surface and repopulate the bare sclera that has been denuded of conjunctiva and exposed to air. It is also a natural substrate for the repopulation of the limbus with normal stem cells that actively divide after the surgical trauma.[34] Its tight junctions prevent the loss of water by evaporation, and its loose connective tissue covers the nerve endings that are bared with the surgical trauma.[9] The normal production of prostaglandins and chemotactic proteins that invite inflammation, white blood cell migration, edema, and pain are thus inhibited. The result is a reduction in postoperative swelling, pain, and recurrence of the pterygium when these membranes are used in the reconstruction of the ocular surface.[5]

Figure 6-12. Role of amniotic membranes in ocular surface reconstruction.

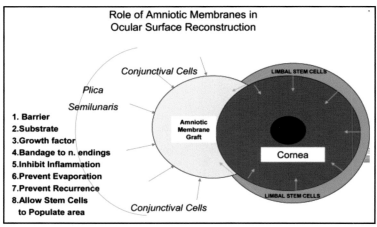

Figure 6-13. The tissue must be rehydrated before use.

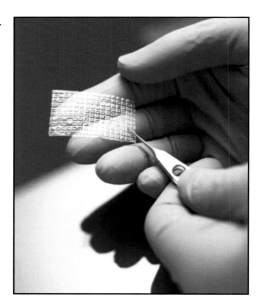

Surgical Principles

- The tissue must be rehydrated before use. If the tissue is transported in alcohol or glycerol, it must be thoroughly rinsed before bringing it into contact with the recipient tissues. If the donor tissue is dehydrated, hydration with BSS suffices prior to grafting onto the recipient bed.

- The epithelial side of the membranes must face upward (Figures 6-12 and 6-13). The graft is designed and transported so that it is easy to identify the epithelial side of the membrane. The AmbioDry membranes have a waffle-shaped pattern that allows identification of the side with the basement membrane, which corresponds to the concave side of the impression. Letters are also printed on the tissue for ease of orientation in the thicker versions of the membrane. Generally, the amniotic membranes have a dull and a shiny side. The shiny side corresponds to the epithelial or basement membrane surface.

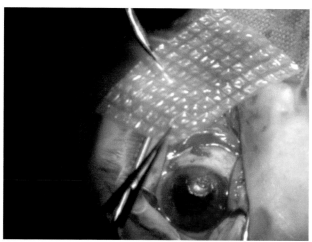

Figure 6-14. Trimming of the amniotic membrane.

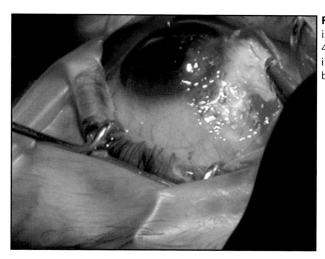

Figure 6-17. Suturing of the graft proceeds in an orderly fashion with placement of 4 cardinal sutures first, followed by the interrupted sutures that are placed in between.

- Trimming of the amniotic membrane should be accomplished before hydration or before application of the membrane to the ocular surface (Figure 6-14).

- Suturing of the graft proceeds in an orderly fashion with the placement of 4 cardinal sutures first, followed by the interrupted sutures that are placed in between (Figure 6-15). It is not necessary to place sutures at the limbal area and the sutures should be always placed so as to imbricate the edge of the donor graft underneath the edge of the recipient conjunctiva.

- If surgical glue is preferred, it is first coated over the scleral bed in a very thin film (Figure 6-16). The donor graft is carefully placed over the cornea and hydrated if necessary. The graft is then advanced over the scleral bed with forceps. The tissue glue acts within seconds and a contact lens is then applied over the cornea.[35]

- If mitomycin-C is to be applied, it must be used prior to the application of the amniotic membrane.[36]

Figure 6-18. Application of surgical glue.

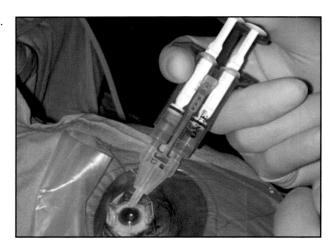

Advantages of the Amniotic Membrane

- Less pain (as no donor site is injured)
- Shorter surgical time
- Faster patient recovery
- Amenable to cover a larger defect
- Saves the donor site for other surgeries such as glaucoma
- Better cosmetic outcome[37]

References

1. Roth A. Plastic repair of conjunctival defects with fetal membranes. *Arch of Ophthalmol.* 1940;23(3): 522-525.
2. Sorsby A, Symons HM. Amniotic membrane grafts in caustic burns of the eye: (burns of the second degree). *Br J of Ophthal.* 1946;30:337-341.
3. John T. Human amniotic membrane transplantation: past, present and future. *Ophthalmol Clin North Am.* 2003;16(1):43-65.
4. Gris O, Güell JL, Lopez-Navidad A, Caballero F, Del Campo Z. Application of the amniotic membrane in ocular surface pathology. *Ann Transplant.* 1999;4:82-84.
5. Cheung PY, Walton JC, Tai HH, Riley SC, Challis JR. Immunocytochemical distribution and localization of 15-hydroxyprostaglandin dehydrogenase in human fetal membranes, decidua, and placenta. *Am J Obstet Gynecol.* 1990;163(5 Pt 1):1445-1449.
6. Rees MC, Di Marzo V, Lopez Bernal A, Tippins JR, Morris HR, Trunbull AC. Leukotriene release by human fetal membranes, placenta and decidua in relation to parturition. *J Endocrinol.* 1988;118(3):497-500.
7. Hao Y, Ma DH, Hwang DG, Kim WS, Zhang F. Identification of antiangiogenic and antiinflammatory proteins in human amniotic membrane. *Cornea.* 2000;19(3):348-352.
8. Kim JC, Tseng SC. The effects on inhibition of corneal neovascularization after human amniotic membrane transplantation in severely damaged rabbit corneas. *Korean J Ophthalmol.* 1995;9(1):32-46.
9. Dua HS, Gomes JA, King AJ, Maharajan VS. The amniotic membrane in ophthalmology. *Surv Ophthalmol.* 2004;49(1):51-77.
10. Batlle JF, Perdomo FJ. Placental membranes as a conjunctival substitute. *Ophthalmology.* 1993;9A:100-107.
11. Dua HS. The conjunctiva in corneal epithelial wound healing. *Br J Ophthalmol.* 1998;82:1407-1411.

12. Batlle JF. Use of amniotic membranes as a conjuntival substitute. Oral presentation at the Annual Resident's Day Meeting of the Bascom Palmer Eye Institute at the Sonesta Beach Hotel in Key Biscayne, Florida, June 1992.

13. Tseng SC, Prabhasawat P, Lee SH. Amniotic membrane transplantation for conjuntival surface reconstruction. *Am J Ophthalmology*. 1997;124:765-774.

14. AmbioDry2 [package insert]. Costa Mesa, CA: OKTO Ophtho; 2007.

15. Aplin JD, Campbell S, Allen TD. The extracellular matrix of human amniotic epithelium: ultrastructure, composition and deposition. *J Cell Sci*. 1985;79:119-136.

16. Franck O, Descargues G, Menguy E. Technique of harvesting and preparation of amniotic membaranes. *J Fr Ophthalmol*. 2000;23:729-734.

17. Van Baare J, Buitenwerf J, Hoekstra MJ, du Pont JS. Virucidal effect of glycerol as used in donor skin preservation. *Burns*. 1994;20:77-80

18. Fukuda K, Chikama T, Nakamura M, Nishida T. Differential distribution of subchains of the basement membrane components type IV collagen and laminin among the amniotic membrane, cornea, and conjunctiva. *Cornea*. 1999;18:73-79.

19. Malak TM, Bell SC. Differential expression of the integrin subunits in human fetal membranes. *J Reprod Fertil*. 1994;102:269-276.

20. Keene DR, Sakai LY, Lunstrum GP, Morris NP, Burgeson RE. Type VII collagen forms an extended network of anchoring fibrils. *J Cell Biol*. 1987;104:611-621.

21. Keelan JA, Sato T, Mitchell MD. Interleukin (IL)-6 and IL-8 production by human amnion: regulation by cytokines, growth factors, glucocorticoids, phorbol esters, and bacterial lipopolysaccharide. *Biol Reprod*. 1997;57:1438-1444.

22. Rote NS, Menon R, Swan KF, Lynden TW. Expression of IL-1 and IL-6 protein and mRNA in amniochorionic membranes. Placenta. 1993;14:A63.

23. Lee SH, Tseng SC. Amniotic membrane transplantation for persistent epithelial defects with ulceration. *Am J Ophthalmol*. 1997;123:303-312.

24. Tseng SC, Li DQ, Ma X, Suppression of transforming growth factor-beta isoforms, TGF-beta receptor type II, and myofibroblast differentiation in cultured human corneal and limbal fibroblast by amniotic membrane matrix. *J Cell Phys Physiol*. 1999;179:325-335.

25. Kubo M, Sonada Y, Muramatsu R, Usui M. Immunogenicity of human amniotic membrane in experimental xenotransplantation. *Invest Ophthalmol Vis Sci*. 2001;42:1539-1546.

26. Grescimanno C, Muhlhauser J, Castellucci M. Immunocytochemichal patterns of carbonic anhydrase isoenzymes in human placenta, cord and membranes. *Placenta*. 1993;14:A11.

27. Tseng SCG, Espana EM, Kawakita T, et al. How does amniotic membrane work? *Ocul Surf*. 2004;2(3):177-187.

28. Kenyon KR, Tseng SCG. Limbal autograft transplantation for ocular surface disorders. *Ophthalmology*. 1989;96:709-723.

29. McCarty C, Fu C, Taylor H. Epidemiology of pterygium in Victoria, Australia. *Br J Ophthalmol*. 2000;84(3):289-292.

30. Lindberg K, Brown ME, Chaves HV, Kenyon KR, Rheinwald JG, In vitro propagation of human ocular surface epithelial cells for transplantation. *Invest Ophthalmol Vis Sci*. 1993;34(9):2672-2679.

31. Danforth D, Hull RW. The microscopic anatomy of the fetal membranes with particular reference to the detailed structure of the amnion. *Am J Obstet Gynecol*. 1958;75:536-550.

32. Van Herendael BJ, Oberti C, Brosens I. Microanatomy of the human amniotic membranes. A light microscopic, transmission, and scanning electron microscopic study. *Am J Obstet Gynecol*. 1978;131(15):872-880.

33. Bourne GL. The microscopic anatomy of the human amnion and chorion. *Am J Obstet Gynecol*. 1960;79:1070-1073.

34. Gabric N, Mravicic I, Dekaris I, Karaman Z, Mitrovic S. Human amniotic membrane in the reconstruction of the ocular surface. *Doc Ophthalmol*. 1999;98:273-283.

35. Jain S, Rastogi A. Evaluation of the outcome of amniotic membrane transplantation for ocular surface reconstruction in symblepharon. *Eye*. 2004;18(12):1251-1257.

36. Ma DH, See LC, Liau SB, Tsai RJ. Amniotic membrane graft for primary pterygium: comparison with conjunctival autograft and topical mitomycin C treatment. *Br J Ophthalmol*. 2000;84:973-978.

37. Tseng, SCG. Pterygium & pinguecula. Ocular Surface Research & Education Foundation Web site. 2011. http://www.osref.org/education_materials/pterygium_and_pinguecula.html. Accessed May 19, 2011.

7

Use of Amniotic Membrane for Conjunctival Reconstruction

Mohamed Abou Shousha, MD; Jane Fishler, MD; and Victor L. Perez, MD

The healing power of the fetal membrane was first reported in modern medicine in 1910. Davis first reported the successful use of amniotic membrane in skin transplantation.[1] Many other reports followed confirming that this membrane promotes re-epithelialization of traumatized skin surfaces, reduces the risk of infection, and markedly decreases pain.[2,3] The idea of using such a tissue to heal the ocular surface seemed appealing to De Rotth, who first introduced it to ophthalmology in 1940.[4] He reported the successful use of amniotic membrane in the treatment of conjunctival epithelial defects after symblepharon lysis surgeries. After a long period of mysterious abandon or under-reporting, this epiphany was revived in the 1990s by Batlle and Perdomo, who seemed to have reminded ophthalmologists of the powers of that membrane, as their report was followed by many other reports of practical uses for amniotic membrane in the management of various ocular surface diseases.[5]

Amniotic membrane, the third innermost layer of the fetal membrane, is essentially a basement membrane graft that contains innumerable growth factors, including basic fibroblast growth factor, epidermal growth factor, hepatocyte growth factor, and transforming growth factor α and β.[6,7] It has been shown to facilitate the proliferation and differentiation of epithelial cells, maintain the original epithelial phenotype, promote goblet cell differentiation, reduce scarring, minimize vascularization, and decrease inflammation.[5,8-10] Moreover, amniotic membrane has proven to be nonimmunogenic as its epithelial cells do not express human leukocyte antigens (HLA)-A, -B, -C, or -DR of β2-microglobulin.[11]

The acknowledgement of all of those properties has prompted the use of amniotic membrane in various conjunctival reconstruction surgeries. It has been used successfully in the management of symptomatic conjunctivochalasis,[12-16] fornix reconstruction after symblepharon lysis,[17-19] acute ocular chemical and thermal burns,[7,20,21] revision of leaking blebs and exposed glaucoma drainage devices,[22-25] primary and recurrent pterygia[26] and conjunctival tumors or other lesions.[27,28]

The purpose of this chapter is to describe the current and described experiences of using amniotic membrane graft for the treatment of disorders that affect the conjunctiva and ocular surface. Indications and surgical techniques will be outlined demonstrating its variable applications in ocular surface reconstruction (Table 7-1).

Hovanesian JA. *Pterygium: Techniques and Technologies for Surgical Success (pp 79-90)*
© 2012 Taylor & Francis Group

TABLE 7-1. THE USE OF AMNIOTIC MEMBRANE GRAFTS IN CONJUNCTIVAL RECONSTRUCTION SURGERIES
1. Symptomatic conjunctivochalasis
2. Fornix reconstruction surgery
3. Acute and chronic chemical and thermal burns
4. Amniotic membrane in the management of glaucoma drainage device exposure and bleb leaks
5. Conjunctival reconstruction after primary and recurrent pterygium excision
6. Conjunctival reconstruction after ocular surface tumors excision

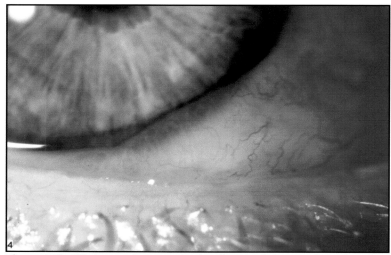

Figure 7-1. Slit lamp photograph showing an inferonasal conjunctivochalasis. Conjunctivochalasis is a redundant, loose, nonedematous bulbar conjunctiva located between the globe and the lower eyelid.

Conjunctivochalasis and Amniotic Membrane Transplantation

Conjunctivochalasis is a redundant, loose, nonedematous bulbar conjunctiva typically located between the globe and the lower eyelid (Figure 7-1). Conjunctivochalasis is not an uncommon condition; however, the trivialization of the condition as a normal senile change has long resulted in overlooking its pathogenic consequences. In the early 1990s, the recognition of the mal-effects of conjunctivochalasis on tear dynamics drew attention and resulted in a new understanding of its pathogenesis and management.[29] We have come to learn that a mild conjunctivochalasis tends to interfere with the tear meniscus and cause or aggravate tear film instability. This gives rise to symptoms characteristic of dry eye, such as burning, foreign body sensation, tiredness upon reading or prolonged use of the eye, and sharp pain and photophobia in its severe forms.[15,30] In moderate conjunctivochalasis, the redundant conjunctival fold can permanently or intermittently block the punctum and cause delayed tear clearance. Delayed tear clearance tends to cause inflammatory symptoms of redness, itching, mucus accumulation, and sticky lids in the morning as well as episodic tearing.[31] In severe cases, exposure-related problems such as nocturnal lagophthalmos and dellen formation could ensue.[12,32]

Conjunctivochalasis tends to be bilateral and typically affects the lower bulbar conjunctiva, more commonly its temporal part. Nevertheless, it can extend to include the superior bulbar conjunctiva and results in a condition that could resemble superior limbal keratoconjunctivitis (SLK).[13,14,33] The similarity between conjunctivochalasis and SLK, in terms of the proposed pathogenesis, raises the question of whether they are 2 different names of the same condition, one located at the superior eyelid and the other along the inferior eyelid. It is noteworthy that superior conjunctivochalasis patients sometimes report ocular pain and light sensitivity, which are not typical for inferior conjunctivochalasis patients.[13]

The first line of treatment of conjunctivochalasis is medical treatment in the form of artificial tears, lubricants, topical steroids, and topical antihistamines. Nevertheless, medical treatment usually does not relieve patients' symptoms, especially in moderate and severe cases. In such a case, surgical removal of the redundant conjunctiva becomes inevitable to control one's symptoms. The reports of inducing complications such as visible conjunctival scarring, cicatricial entropion of the lower lid, retraction of the lower fornix, restricted motility, or corneal problems in the course of the surgical management of conjunctivochalasis have long discouraged surgeons to operate upon mild and moderate cases.[16,32] The introduction of amniotic membrane to ocular surface surgery with its well-acknowledged anti-inflammatory, antiscarring, and antiangiogenic actions and its growth-promoting effects have encouraged definitive surgical treatment in patients who failed to respond to medical treatment.

Amniotic membrane acts as a free graft after excision of redundant conjunctiva. It can be fixed in place using sutures. The downsides of using sutures, beside prolongation of the operating time, are postoperative discomfort and suture-related complications such as abscesses, granuloma formation, and giant papillary conjunctivitis. The use of fibrin glue to fix the amniotic membrane in place with no sutures has optimized surgery by eliminating the aforementioned complications, shortening the operating time, and minimizing patients' postoperative discomfort.

The surgery is done under topical anesthesia. A 7-0 Vicryl traction suture (Ethicon, Inc, Somerville, NJ) is placed at the 6 o'clock position of the cornea 1 mm from the limbus to rotate the eye upward and allow for proper exposure. Grasping the conjunctiva with a forceps and tenting it upward will demonstrate the redundant conjunctiva. This redundant conjunctiva is then excised in an arc-shaped fashion. Hemostasis is achieved using a diathermy. The 2 solutions of the fibrin glue are applied to the edges of the excised conjunctival to fix it to the underlying sclera and, at the same time, to control any blood leakage. Amniotic membrane is laid on the sclera with the stromal surface down and fashioned to cover the area of the excised conjunctiva. Half of the membrane is folded over onto the other half to expose the stromal surface. The thrombin solution is applied to the scleral surface while the fibrinogen solution is applied to the stromal surface of the amniotic membrane. The membrane is flipped back to cover the bare sclera and a muscle hook is used to spread the fibrin glue under the amniotic membrane. These steps are then repeated for the other half of the membrane (Figures 7-2 and 7-3).

Superior conjunctivochalasis can be surgically managed similarly to inferior conjunctivochalasis by excising an arc of the superior loose conjunctiva and covering the bare sclera with an amniotic membrane. Kheirkhah et al have proposed a different surgical technique based on their hypothesis that looseness of superior bulbar

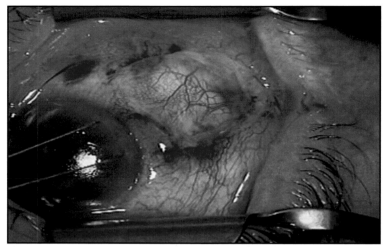

Figure 7-2. An inferonasal conjunctivochalasis. The redundant inferonasal conjunctiva is excised in an arc-shaped fashion. An amniotic membrane graft is glued over the bare sclera.

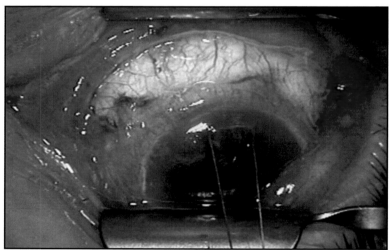

Figure 7-3. An inferior conjunctivochalasis. The amniotic membrane acts as a free graft covering the bare sclera after excision of the redundant inferior conjunctiva. Fibrin glue is used to fix the amniotic membrane in place.

conjunctiva is caused by the lack of adhesion between the conjunctiva and the sclera due to the loss or the lack of Tenon's tissue, rather than simple redundancy of conjunctiva.[13] Their technique consists of the transplantation of amniotic membrane with fibrin glue or sutures to replace the missing Tenon's tissue. This will reinforce the adhesion of the remaining Tenon's tissue with the sclera without resection or recession of the conjunctival tissue.

Favorable results that were achieved using amniotic membrane grafts have encouraged more definitive surgical management of symptomatic cases of conjunctivochalasis.[5,15,16,32,34] Complications of conjunctival wound healing, such as visible conjunctival scarring, cicatricial entropion of the lower lid, retraction of the lower fornix, restricted motility, or corneal problems have largely disappeared from the literature after employing amniotic membrane grafts in conjunctivochalasis management. The use of fibrin glue instead of sutures has further optimized surgical outcomes by eliminating suture-related complications such as granuloma and minimizing postoperative inflammation and discomfort.

Role of Amniotic Membrane Transplantation in Fornix Reconstruction Surgery

Symblepharon, or shortening of the fornices and their obliteration by fibrous tissue, can impose major morbidities on the ocular surface and—in its severest forms—could ultimately lead to failure of the ocular surface and corneal blindness. Interruption of the tear flow and spread is a common consequence and can result in dry eye. It can also lead to repeated blink-related ocular trauma from the resultant irregular tarsal surface, cicatricial entropion, or misdirected lashes that would impose deleterious damage to the cornea. Finally, patients may also have limitation of Bell's phenomenon as well as restricting ocular motility resulting in diplopia.[17,35] Several etiological factors are implicated in the development of symblepharon. They include infections, cicatrizing conjunctival autoimmune diseases, drugs, chemical burns, or previous surgeries.

Etiological factors such as active ocular cicatricial pemphigoid or trachoma infection must be controlled first before any attempt can be made to interfere surgically. If those factors remain untreated, surgery will carry a high risk of recurrence. Several techniques have been reported for the surgical correction of symblepharon. All share the essential steps of lysis of the cicatrix followed by reconstruction of the ocular surface with autologous conjunctival graft, amniotic membrane graft, and/or oral mucosal grafts.[19,36,37] Adjunctive measures include applying intraoperative mitomycin-C (MMC), anchoring sutures to secure the released conjunctiva deep into the fornix, inserting a conformer, and implanting a silicone sheet.[35,38]

The successful use of amniotic membrane grafts in fornix reconstruction is based on a proper understanding of the properties and capabilities of amniotic membrane grafts. Kheirkhah et al reported that the use of amniotic membrane graft for fornix reconstruction can achieve a high success rate only if the length of the residual recessed conjunctiva was at least sufficient to cover the tarsal conjunctiva.[17] Otherwise, in more severe cases, the success rate was not satisfactory. Those severe cases benefited from the combination of amniotic membrane, oral mucosal, and autologous conjunctival grafts (Figures 7-4 and 7-5). Severe symblepharon is almost always associated with severe dry eye, and the prognosis for the use of amniotic membrane grafts in such cases is very poor. Jain and Rastogi reported that fornix reconstruction using amniotic membrane graft in cases with severe dry eye had a 100% failure rate.[18] The poor performance of amniotic membrane grafts in such cases can be explained by proper understanding of the structure and nature of amniotic membrane. Despite all its anti-inflammatory and growth factors, it is still primarily a basement membrane that will promote epithelial cell growth over it and thus act as a substrate, but not a substitute, for conjunctiva.[18]

Amniotic membrane transplantation (AMT) could be used to successfully reconstruct the conjunctiva after lysis of symblepharon in mild cases where the ocular surface still has "healthy" characteristics such as good lubrication and lack of severe scarring. In severe cases, amniotic membrane graft alone would not yield satisfactory results. AMT in such cases should be an adjunctive step rather than the definitive management plan.

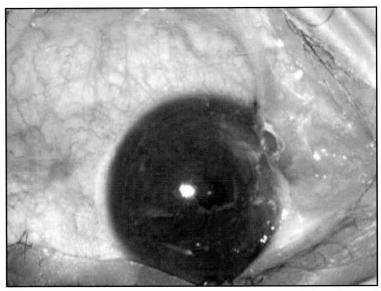

Figure 7-4. Recurrent pterygium with symblepharon to medial canthus and upper and lower eyelids. Symblepharon resulted in an esotropic restrictive strabismus with complete loss of abduction and diplopia in primary gaze.

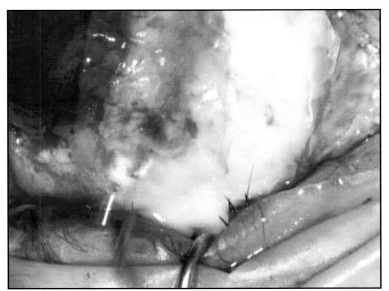

Figure 7-5. Immediate postoperative photograph of the patient in Figure 7-4. After identifying and hooking the medial rectus muscle, the recurrent pterygium and the subconjunctival fibrous tissue were completely excised. Adhesions to the muscle sheath were released. Orbital septum reconstruction was performed. MMC (0.04%) was applied for 2 minutes to the edges of the residual conjunctiva. An autologous conjunctival graft was glued to the nasal limbus. Sutures were only used to secure the limbal side of the graft as no glue was used over the cornea. Care was taken to incorporate a keratolimbal graft to the conjunctival graft. An oral mucosal graft was glued over the muscle and bare sclera, reconstructing the upper and lower fornices. An amniotic membrane graft was then glued over the conjunctiva, oral grafts, and the nasal limbus.

Amniotic Membrane
Transplant in Chemical Burns

Chemical burn of the ocular surface can have deleterious effects on the eye globe. It usually results in limbal stem cell destruction that can lead to chronic corneal inflammation, neovascularization, conjunctivalization, and persistent epithelial defects that can ultimately lead to corneal blindness. Conjunctival epithelium could also be affected by the destruction of goblet cells, which may induce keratinization, scarring, and symblepharon formation.

The main goal of restoring vision in such patients is recreating the anatomic and physiologic structure of the ocular surface with reconstruction of the corneal and conjunctival epithelium.[39] Several surgical techniques have been previously attempted for ocular surface reconstruction after chemical burns such as the simple excision of the fibrous tissue followed by a corneal transplant. Those techniques, however, were not successful due to the recurrence of the fibrovascular pannus.[40] Combining limbal stem cell with AMT has been shown to yield the best reported results. Limbal stem cell transplantation is crucial to restoration of the corneal epithelium, while an amniotic membrane is used to recreate the appropriate environment for conjunctival epithelium restoration. The microenvironment created by the amniotic membrane promotes a better survival of the transplanted limbal stem cells and increases the success rate of ocular surface reconstruction.

Amniotic Membrane Transplantation in Acute Chemical Burns

The prognosis of an eye with a chemical burn depends not only on the severity of the damage induced by the burn, but also on the rapidity and the mode of treatment. The use of AMT as a biological patch in cases with acute chemical burns has been shown to aid in re-epithelialization, reduction of inflammation, pain relief, visual improvement, and preservation of ocular surface integrity.[20] The anti-inflammatory effects of AMT mediated by antiproteases and suppression of interleukin-1 (IL-1) release seems to prevent patients from experiencing visual loss due to aggressive postinjury scarring. As a result, symblepharon is also a rare complication in those patients.[20,21]

In severe cases of an acute chemical burn, AMT is used to cover the entire ocular surface. After débridement of necrotic conjunctival tissue, AMT is anchored to the upper and lower lid margins. It is secured over the ocular surface using episcleral bites of interrupted 9-0 or 10-0 Vicryl sutures. Double-armed horizontal mattress sutures with external ties over the skin are placed in the upper and lower fornices of the lid to prevent symblepharon formation. However, in less severe cases, AMT may be sutured only to the damaged areas of the ocular surface.[21,41] Nevertheless, it is important to note that those favorable results are limited to cases with mild and moderate burns. In cases with severe chemical burns, AMT has not been shown to yield favorable results. Limbal stem deficiency is not prevented by the temporary AMT patch and thus its use in cases with severe chemical burns may be inadequate.

Chronic Chemical Burn and Limbal Stem Cell Deficiency

Gomes et al described 2 groups of patients postchemical injury: those with partial limbal stem cell deficiency (PLD) and those with total limbal stem cell deficiency (TLD).[39] The group of patients with PLD had successful ocular surface reconstruction with preserved AMT alone, while the second group with TLD was treated with AMT and limbal stem cell transplantation. Surgical procedure involved removing the conjunctival epithelium with fibrous tissue covering the cornea 3 to 4 mm posterior to the limbus, symblepharon dissection, and placement of the amniotic membrane over the created defect. In those cases with TLD, limbal stem cell transplantation was also performed. Surgical success was favorable in cases of PLD. On the other hand, the results were not as favorable as in the TLD group, which can most likely be attributed to the more complex nature of those cases.

In cases with PLD, abnormally vascularized epithelium and pannus should be excised, leaving normal limbal and corneal epithelium intact. AMT is tailored to cover the created defect with the basement membrane up. The orientation of the membrane can be confirmed intraoperatively by touching it with a Weck-cel sponge (Medtronic, Minneapolis, MN), thus demonstrating the stickiness of the stromal side of the membrane.[21] The membrane is secured to the edges of the corneal defect with interrupted 10-0 nylon sutures. If a wide limbal area must be covered, the membrane can be secured with an episcleral pursing running 9-0 or 10-0 Vicryl suture. Symblepharon lysis and fornix reconstruction should be combined with the AMT as needed. In cases with TLD, AMT is used in conjunction with limbal stem cell and conjunctival grafts and serves as a biological bandage covering the entire surgical site.

AMT is useful in mild to moderate cases of acute chemical injury because it promotes epithelialization, reduces surface inflammation, and decreases vascularization and scarring formation in this group of patients, although the merits of using AMT in severe cases is questionable. Patients with chronic changes from chemical injury may benefit from AMT implantation in conjunction with a limbal stem cell transplant to promote an inflammation-free environment and provide the basal membrane onto which the stem cells can migrate and proliferate.[42]

Amniotic Membrane Transplantation in Glaucoma Surgeries With Conjunctival Complications

Amniotic Membrane in the Management of Glaucoma Drainage Device Exposure

Glaucoma drainage devices are frequently used in the management of uncontrolled glaucoma refractory to full medical therapy. One of the complications of this surgical procedure is melting the overlying sclera or bovine pericardial patch with exposure of the tube through the conjunctiva. This occurs in 2% to 7% of patients undergoing this surgery.[22] As a result, patients can experience significant discomfort and may be at an increased risk of developing intraocular infection and endophthalmitis. When trying to repair the exposed tube, one has to replace the scleral patch and once again cover it with the remaining conjunctiva. Primary closures, as well as conjunctival autografts, have been used to repair this problem. However, in patients with multiple previous ocular surgeries such as trabeculectomies, pterygium excisions, and multiple placements of glaucoma drainage devices, conjunctival closure may be more challenging. Conjunctival tissue in such patients is more fragile and may be strongly adherent to the underlying scar tissue. As a result, amniotic membrane has been used in the management of this complication.

Amniotic membrane can be used to repair exposed tubes since its basement membrane will promote epithelialization and adhesion while the stromal bed can help reduce inflammation, vascularization, and fibrosis.[23] Ainsworth et al proposed a method of a 2-layered amniotic membrane patch graft to repair the defect.[22] The conjunctiva was first reflected around the exposed tube and a new full-thickness scleral patch was secured to the tube. The first layer of the amniotic membrane is then placed over the sclera patch with the epithelial side up. The membrane size is cut larger than the actual defect since it can be tucked under the free edges of the remaining conjunctiva and will provide a substrate for epithelial cell migration to close the defect. Finally, a second layer of the conjunctiva is placed over the defect, epithelial side down. Again, the membrane is cut larger than the conjunctival defect and acts as a bandage to the first layer below. It falls off several weeks after its placement. Each layer of the amniotic membrane is secured to the eye with 10-0 nylon sutures. Papdaki et al reported another case report of a tube exposure where an artificial dura was used as a patch.[23] In the process of repair, the dura was removed and the tube was covered with a single layer of an amniotic membrane sutured to the sclera and the remaining conjunctiva. Both methods successfully repaired the glaucoma drainage device exposure.

Increased tension of the conjunctiva over the tube, mechanical breakdown, ischemia, and necrosis all cause conjunctival erosion. It is important to evaluate patients carefully for these risk factors and keep AMT as an option in patients with multiple episodes of tube exposure.

Amniotic Membrane in the Management of Bleb Leaks

Glaucoma-filtering surgery is commonly used in patients with progressive glaucoma despite maximal medical management. Leakage of aqueous fluid from a conjunctival filtering bleb is one of the complications of this surgery. This has become especially frequent due to the application of MMC, which is used to reduce fibrosis and scarring in the area of the bleb. Reported rates of bleb leaks in such patients range from 3.7% to 13.6 %.[43]

Bleb leaks are considered an emergency because they may lead to more severe complications such as hypotony, maculopathy, choroidal detachments, and endophthalmitis. Several methods have been used to repair bleb leaks, including advancement of the conjunctival flap, placing tissue adhesive over the area of the leak, or suturing a free conjunctival graft over the leak. These techniques can be challenging in patients with large blebs and can result in failure of filtration due to external scarring.[44] Superior conjunctival advancement can also be associated with ptosis and diplopia due to interference with the levator-superior rectus complex. As a result, amniotic membrane has been used in many cases to repair this frequent complication.

Budenz et al compared 2 groups of patients with filtering blebs.[44] Eyes were randomized to have bleb excision followed by conjunctival advancement versus AMT. After a mean follow-up of 19 months, nearly 50% of the amniotic membrane repairs failed primarily due to bleb leaks, compared with zero failures in the conjunctival advancement group. However, since then, new techniques have been proposed and more favorable results have been reported. Among the new techniques are no bleb excision, placing AMT underneath the conjunctiva, and double-layered AMT techniques.[24] Kitagawa et al developed a technique using a hyper-dry amniotic membrane patch for bleb leaks.[43] The dried amniotic membrane was cut to an appropriate size with scissors, and tissue adhesive was used to secure the membrane with the epithelial side placed over the area of the leak. No recurrence of bleb leaks was noted in 26 months of follow up. This technique is especially useful in patients with avascular blebs in which suturing may induce a new leak from the sutured sites.

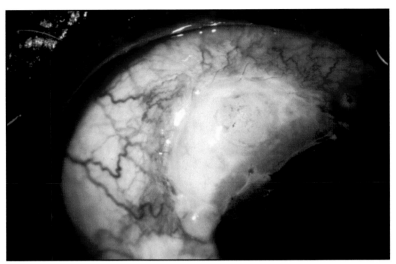

Figure 7-6. Amniotic membrane repair of glaucoma bleb leak. After complete excision of the old filtering bleb, amniotic membrane was used to cover the resultant conjunctival defect. The amniotic membrane is sutured to the peripheral cornea using interrupted sutures and to the underside of the surrounding conjunctiva using a continuous running suture. (Reprinted with permission of Francisco E. Fantes, MD.)

Amniotic membrane may be a useful alternate technique to repair a posttrabeculectomy bleb leak, especially in cases where there is inadequate conjunctiva for a conjunctival advancement, avascular blebs, or in those with forniceal foreshortening and preoperative diplopia (Figure 7-6).

Conclusion

Management of conjunctival scarring, fibrosis, and inflammation is not trivial. Even though the treatment of conjunctival diseases that lead to inflammation, fibrosis, and scarring are complex, the use of amniotic membrane grafts has proven to be effective and has achieved favorable results in many conjunctival reconstruction surgeries. Amniotic membrane is essentially a basement membrane graft that contains crucial antiscarring, antiangiogenic, and growth-promoting factors. Understanding its merits and limitations will certainly lead to its successful employment in reconstructing the ocular surface.

References

1. Davis JW. Skin transplantation with a review of 550 cases at the Johns Hopkins Hospital. *Johns Hopkins Med J.* 1910;15:307-396.
2. Sabella N. Use of fetal membranes in skin grafting. *Med Records NY.* 1913;83:478-480.
3. Bennett JP, Matthews R, Faulk WP. Treatment of chronic ulceration of the legs with human amnion. *Lancet.* 1980;1:1153-1156.
4. De Rotth A. Plastic repair of conjunctival defects with fetal membranes. *Arch Ophthal.* 1940;23:522-525.

5. Dua HS, Gomes JA, King AJ, Maharajan VS. The amniotic membrane in ophthalmology. *Surv Ophthalmol.* 2004;49:51-77.
6. Koizumi NJ, Inatomi TJ, Sotozono CJ, Fullwood NJ, Quantock AJ, Kinoshita S. Growth factor mRNA and protein in preserved human amniotic membrane. *Curr Eye Res.* 2000;20:173-177.
7. Shimazaki J, Yang HY, Tsubota K. Amniotic membrane transplantation for ocular surface reconstruction in patients with chemical and thermal burns. *Ophthalmology.* 1997;104:2068-2076.
8. Prabhasawat P, Tseng SC. Impression cytology study of epithelial phenotype of ocular surface reconstructed by preserved human amniotic membrane. *Arch Ophthalmol.* 1997;115:1360-1367.
9. Meller D, Dabul V, Tseng SC. Expansion of conjunctival epithelial progenitor cells on amniotic membrane. *Exp Eye Res.* 2002;74:537-545.
10. Kim JC, Tseng SC. Transplantation of preserved human amniotic membrane for surface reconstruction in severely damaged rabbit corneas. *Cornea.* 1995;14:473-484.
11. Adinolfi M, Akle CA, McColl I, et al. Expression of HLA antigens, beta 2-microglobulin and enzymes by human amniotic epithelial cells. *Nature.* 1982;295:325-327.
12. Meller D, Tseng SC. Conjunctivochalasis: literature review and possible pathophysiology. *Surv Ophthalmol.* 1998;43:225-232.
13. Kheirkhah A, Casas V, Esquenazi S, et al. New surgical approach for superior conjunctivochalasis. *Cornea.* 2007;26:685-691.
14. Yokoi N, Komuro A, Maruyama K, Tsuzuki M, Miyajima S, Kinoshita S. New surgical treatment for superior limbic keratoconjunctivitis and its association with conjunctivochalasis. *Am J Ophthalmol.* 2003;135:303-308.
15. Meller D, Maskin SL, Pires RT, Tseng SC. Amniotic membrane transplantation for symptomatic conjunctivochalasis refractory to medical treatments. *Cornea.* 2000;19:796-803.
16. Serrano F, Mora LM. Conjunctivochalasis: a surgical technique. *Ophthalmic Surg.* 1989;20:883-884.
17. Kheirkhah A, Blanco G, Casas V, Hayashida Y, Raju VK, Tseng SC. Surgical strategies for fornix reconstruction based on symblepharon severity. *Am J Ophthalmol.* 2008;146:266-275.
18. Jain S, Rastogi A. Evaluation of the outcome of amniotic membrane transplantation for ocular surface reconstruction in symblepharon. *Eye (Lond).* 2004;18:1251-1257.
19. Solomon A, Espana EM, Tseng SC. Amniotic membrane transplantation for reconstruction of the conjunctival fornices. *Ophthalmology.* 2003;110:93-100.
20. Kobayashi A, Shirao Y, Yoshita T, et al. Temporary amniotic membrane patching for acute chemical burns. *Eye (Lond).* 2003;17:149-158.
21. Meller D, Pires RT, Mack RJ, et al. Amniotic membrane transplantation for acute chemical or thermal burns. *Ophthalmology.* 2000;107:980-989.
22. Ainsworth G, Rotchford A, Dua HS, King AJ. A novel use of amniotic membrane in the management of tube exposure following glaucoma tube shunt surgery. *Br J Ophthalmol.* 2006;90:417-419.
23. Papadaki TG, Siganos CS, Zacharopoulos IP, Panteleontidis V, Charissis SK. Human amniotic membrane transplantation for tube exposure after glaucoma drainage device implantation. *J Glaucoma.* 2007;16:171-172.
24. Rauscher FM, Barton K, Budenz DL, Feuer WJ, Tseng SC. Long-term outcomes of amniotic membrane transplantation for repair of leaking glaucoma filtering blebs. *Am J Ophthalmol.* 2007;143:1052-1054.
25. Kee C, Hwang JM. Amniotic membrane graft for late-onset glaucoma filtering leaks. *Am J Ophthalmol.* 2002;133:834-835.
26. Ti SE, Tseng SC. Management of primary and recurrent pterygium using amniotic membrane transplantation. *Curr Opin Ophthalmol.* 2002;13:204-212.
27. Mehta M, Waner M, Fay A. Amniotic membrane grafting in the management of conjunctival vascular malformations. *Ophthal Plast Reconstr Surg.* 2009;25:371-375.
28. Paridaens D, Beekhuis H, van Den Bosch W, Remeyer L, Melles G. Amniotic membrane transplantation in the management of conjunctival malignant melanoma and primary acquired melanosis with atypia. *Br J Ophthalmol.* 2001;85:658-661.
29. Grene RB. Conjunctival pleating and keratoconjunctivitis sicca. *Cornea.* 1991;10:367-368.
30. Lemp MA. Report of the national eye institute/industry workshop on clinical trials in dry eyes. *CLAO J.* 1995;21:221-232.
31. Prabhasawat P, Tseng SC. Frequent association of delayed tear clearance in ocular irritation. *Br J Ophthalmol.* 1998;82:666-675.
32. Liu D. Conjunctivochalasis. A cause of tearing and its management. *Ophthal Plast Reconstr Surg.* 1986;2:25-28.
33. Mimura T, Usui T, Yamagami S, et al. Subconjunctival hemorrhage and conjunctivochalasis. *Ophthalmology.* 2009;116:1880-1886.
34. Di Pascuale MA, Espana EM, Kawakita T, Tseng SC. Clinical characteristics of conjunctivochalasis with or without aqueous tear deficiency. *Br J Ophthalmol.* 2004;88:388-392.

35. Tseng SC, Di Pascuale MA, Liu DT, Gao YY, Baradaran-Rafii A. Intraoperative mitomycin C and amniotic membrane transplantation for fornix reconstruction in severe cicatricial ocular surface diseases. *Ophthalmology.* 2005;112:896-903.
36. Kaufman HE, Thomas EL. Prevention and treatment of symblepharon. *Am J Ophthalmol.* 1979;88:419-423.
37. Ballen PH. Mucous membrane grafts in chemical (lye) burns. *Am J Ophthalmol.* 1963;55:302-312.
38. Choy AE, Asbell RL, Taterka HB. Symblepharon repair using a silicone sheet implant. *Ann Ophthalmol.* 1977;9:197-204.
39. Gomes JA, dos Santos MS, Cunha MC, Mascaro VL, Barros Jde N, de Sousa LB. Amniotic membrane transplantation for partial and total limbal stem cell deficiency secondary to chemical burn. *Ophthalmology.* 2003;110:466-473.
40. Tseng SC, Prabhasawat P, Barton K, Gray T, Meller D. Amniotic membrane transplantation with or without limbal allografts for corneal surface reconstruction in patients with limbal stem cell deficiency. *Arch Ophthalmol.* 1998;116:431-441.
41. Brown AL. Lime burns of the eye: use of rabbit peritoneum to prevent severe delayed effects: experimental studies and report of cases. *Arch Ophthal.* 1941;26:754-769.
42. Ucakhan OO, Koklu G, Firat E. Nonpreserved human amniotic membrane transplantation in acute and chronic chemical eye injuries. *Cornea.* 2002;21:169-172.
43. Kitagawa K, Yanagisawa S, Watanabe K, et al. A hyperdry amniotic membrane patch using a tissue adhesive for corneal perforations and bleb leaks. *Am J Ophthalmol.* 2009;148:383-389.
44. Budenz DL, Barton K, Tseng SC. Amniotic membrane transplantation for repair of leaking glaucoma filtering blebs. *Am J Ophthalmol.* 2000;130:580-588.

8

Pterygium Excision and Placement of Amniotic Membrane Grafts

Hyung Cho, MD and Roy S. Chuck, MD, PhD

More than a hundred techniques for pterygium surgery have been described over the past several centuries because of concern over recurrence. Corneal specialists favor 1 of 2 approaches for surgical removal: simple excision with primary closure after controlled application of mitomycin-C (MMC) intraoperatively or excision followed by free conjunctival autograft.[1] The use of the antimetabolite MMC was a widely used alternative, but its value has become more limited due to its potential long-term toxic effects.[1] Successful results have been reported in various studies with the conjunctival autograft technique. However, this technique has 2 important limitations: it is difficult to close the large conjunctival defects, and there is a need to reserve conjunctiva for glaucoma surgery with a filtering bleb (which may be required in the future). Moreover, in cases where the conjunctiva is scarred from previous surgery for pterygium, alternative surgical techniques must be used.[2]

These problems necessitated the development of amniotic membrane for pterygium surgery. This chapter will discuss the history of the amniotic membrane, the types of amniotic membrane in use, fibrin glue in pterygium surgery, surgical technique, and some of the limitations of the amniotic membrane.

History of Amniotic Membrane Transplantation

The amniotic membrane, or amnion, is the innermost layer of the placenta and is derived from fetal membranes. The inner amniotic membrane is made of a single layer of amnion cells fixed to collagen-rich mesenchyme, 6 to 8 cell layers thick and loosely attached to chorion. It is composed of 3 layers: a single epithelial layer, a thick basement membrane, and avascular stroma.[3] The epithelium and stroma are endowed with a number of cytokines and growth factors, key among which are transforming growth factor beta (TGF-β)[4] and epidermal growth factor.[5] The exact mechanism of action is not clearly defined, but it is widely accepted to act as a substrate in most instances,

Hovanesian JA. *Pterygium: Techniques and Technologies for Surgical Success (pp 91-100)*
© 2012 Taylor & Francis Group

which is very conducive to epithelial cell migration and attachment. Its biological constituents as mentioned above also contribute to its beneficial effect.[6] Human amniotic membrane is believed to be nonimmunogenic. Antibodies or cell-mediated immune response to amniotic membrane have not been demonstrated, suggesting low antigenicity. Therefore, the use of systemic immunosuppressives in amniotic membrane transplantation (AMT) may not be required.[7]

The first reported use of fetal membranes in skin transplantation was by Davis in 1910.[8] The first use of AMT in ophthalmology was by De Rotth in 1940, who reported partial success in the treatment of conjunctival epithelial defects after symblepharon.[9] Little else regarding amniotic membrane appeared in the ophthalmic literature until 1995, when Kim and Tseng used AMT for ocular surface reconstruction of severely damaged corneas in a rabbit model.[10] They showed that 40% of corneas with total limbal deficiency can be reconstructed by replacing the conjunctivalized surface with a preserved human amniotic membrane.

Since that experimental study, preserved human amniotic membrane has been advocated for the management of many ocular surface disorders, such as persistent corneal epithelial defects, ocular surface reconstruction for conjunctival neoplasm or scarring, chemical or thermal burns, advanced ocular cicatricial pemphigoid, Stevens-Johnson syndrome, corneal scarring following excimer laser photoablation, prevention of trabeculectomy failure, and coverage of conjunctival defects after pterygium excision.[11] The CPT code for AMT for ocular surface reconstruction is 65780. As of February 2010, there are close to 800 peer-reviewed publications for the ocular use of amniotic membrane, highlighting novel and therapeutic applications.

AMT has been shown to suppress fibrosis when used for pterygium surgery. Tseng et al[12] demonstrated that the TGF-β signaling pathway in fibroblasts was strongly suppressed when in contact with the stromal side of the amniotic membrane. Because TGF-βs are potent fibrogenic growth factors, suppression of the signaling pathway has an antifibrosis effect. In addition, the amniotic membrane has an anti-inflammatory effect, which may contribute to proper postoperative wound healing.[13] Because amniotic membrane grafts have virtually no limitation in terms of size, fibrotic tissue can be extensively excised. This advantage may also contribute to favorable surgical outcomes.

Types and Methods of Preservation of Amniotic Membrane

One placenta provides sufficient amniotic membrane for 20 to 30 ophthalmic transplants. Many methods for preserving and storing amniotic membranes have been described, but 2 important methods are in vogue. In its freeze-dried form, it is known as AmbioDry (IOP Ophthalmics, Costa Mesa, CA; Figure 8-1), and it is known as Amniograft (BioTissue Inc, Miami, FL) in its cryopreserved form (Figure 8-2). Preservation by freezing (Amniograft) at -80°C is a common mode of preservation before use. This involves the use of 2 types of solutions: either phosphate-buffered saline (PBS) in dimethyl sulfoxide (DMSO) or in Eagle's minimum essential medium (MEM) with glycerol.[14] Amniotic membrane is harvested during elective cesarian section from consenting maternal donors, who are seronegative for Hepatitis B and C virus, syphilis, and human immunodeficiency virus (HIV). Under sterile conditions, the placental membrane is washed in a balanced salt solution (BSS) to remove clots

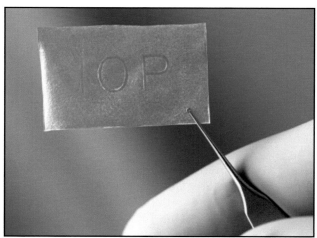

Figure 8-1. AmbioDry. (Reprinted with permission from IOP Ophthalmics, Inc, Costa Mesa, CA, www.iopinc.com.)

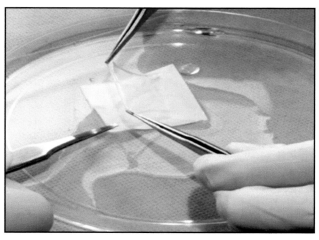

Figure 8-2. Amniograft, www.biotissue.com. (Reprinted with permission of Hosam Sheha, MD, PhD.)

and debris. The membrane is then bathed in a cocktail of antimicrobial medium for 24 hours, followed by a second wash in BSS. Subsequently, the amnion is separated from the chorion and divided into pieces measuring approximately 2 cm by 2 cm and mounted, stromal side down, onto nitrocellulose cards. The membrane is then placed in a plastic container, and stored in 50% glycerol at -80°C for up to 2 years. Serological tests are repeated on the maternal donor 6 months after delivery before its release for clinical use.[15] The tissue in Amniograft is ready for transplantation immediately after removing it from the carrier paper without the need for rehydration.

AmbioDry is electron-beam sterilized and is free standing, without attachment to nitrocellulose paper. Because it is stored dry, it can be kept at room temperature with no freezing or refrigeration required. The graft can be applied to the surgical site and rehydrated with sterile saline within minutes and without thawing or soaking.

Human amniotic membrane has been reported to produce various immunosuppressive cytokines such as interleukin 4 (IL-4), IL-10, and TGF-β1 and -β2.[16-18] Although the exact mechanism is still unclear, the immunosuppressive properties of cryopreserved amniotic membrane have been demonstrated by mouse T-cell suppression.[19] A study testing the immunosuppressive properties of dry human amniotic membrane found that it is indeed immunosuppressive and that membrane with intact amniotic epithelium (AmbioDry 2) was more immunosuppressive than dry amniotic membrane without epithelium (AmbioDry 1).[20] AmbioDry 5, the newer third-generation amniotic membrane, is thicker at 110 µm (as compared to the 40-µm thick AmbioDry 2). It is thicker because it retains additional collagen matrices from the placental interface during processing.[21]

AmbioDry was found to maintain desirable elastic characteristics in transition from a dry to rehydrated state and thus may provide an easy-to-manipulate transplant tissue. In comparison, frozen Amniograft required greater forces to rupture.[22] The choice of either product depends upon an individual surgeon's comfort using either material.

In many parts of the developing world, fresh, unpreserved membrane (within days or weeks of donation) is still used. In the United States and Western countries, however, fresh membrane is not used because of legislation requiring that the membrane be adequately screened for HIV contamination. To this end, the donors are tested at the time of delivery and 6 months later (to cover the window period of infection). All processed membranes are stored in quarantine until the second test is performed and reported negative.

Adjunctive Use of Fibrin Glue in Pterygium Surgery

Traditionally during pterygium surgery, the conjunctival autografts are secured in place with either absorbable or nonabsorbable sutures. Suture placement may significantly add to operative time. In addition, sutures are usually associated with significant postoperative discomfort and inflammation. Fibrin glue is a 2-component tissue adhesive that mimics natural fibrin formation and can be used to attach either conjunctival autografts or amniotic membranes without the use of sutures. The use of fibrin glue during pterygium surgery was first described by Cohen and McDonald in 1993.[23] Because of its biological and biodegradable properties, fibrin-based adhesives may be used under a superficial covering layer (eg, conjunctiva, amniotic membrane) without inducing inflammation.[24] It has been used in ophthalmology for indications including lamellar keratoplasty, glaucoma surgery, and strabismus wound closure.[25-27]

There are currently 2 main types of fibrin glue on the US market: Tisseel VH (Baxter Healthcare Corp, Deerfield, IL)[28] and Evicel (Ethicon Inc, Somerville, NJ).[29] Tisseel is a human-fibrin tissue adhesive consisting of a combination of fibrinogen and thrombin, which forms an adhesive fibrin network when mixed. Tisseel is commercially available and is used in cardiovascular stent surgery; orthopedics; neurosurgery; plastic surgery; and ear, nose, and throat surgery.[30-32] The glue has 2 components: a sealant protein, which is a freeze-dried powder composed of human fibrinogen, fibronectin, plasminogen, and factor XIII reconstituted in a bovine aprotinin solution; and sealant setting, a solution composed of human thrombin reconstituted in a calcium chloride solution. When the solutions interact, through the action of thrombin, the fibrinopeptides are broken down to fibrin monomers by utilizing the last step of the blood coagulation cascade. These monomers aggregate by cross-linking, leading to formation of a fibrin clot.[33] The source of the thrombin and fibrinogen in Tisseel is pooled human sera. Donors are tested, and retested after a 3-month interval, for viral infections including hepatitis B and C, HIV, and human parvovirus. Vapor heating adds another measure of safety to the product. In more than 10 million uses of Tisseel, there have been no reports of infection with hepatitis, HIV, or bovine spongiform encephalitis (mad cow disease).[1]

Evicel[29] is the only all-human, plasma-derived fibrin sealant commercially available in the United States. Evicel was initially approved for general hemostasis in surgery, when control of bleeding by standard surgical techniques is ineffective or impractical. Unlike Tisseel, it does not contain aprotinin (a bovine lung tissue-derived component), which has been associated with adverse health effects such as an increased risk of renal failure, stroke, myocardial infarction, and mortality.[34]

Studies have evaluated the efficacy and safety of fibrin glue in pterygium surgery with conjunctival autografting and found that fibrin glue provided adequate adhesion of conjunctival grafts to the ocular surface similar to those reported in the literature for sutured grafts and without significant complications.[35] A recent retrospective study on a large cohort suggested that pterygium surgery with fibrin glue leads to significantly lower recurrence rates when compared with the use of sutures.[36]

Pterygium Surgery With Amniotic Membrane

An ideal pterygium surgery should achieve 3 principal goals: a low recurrence rate, lack of complications, and a satisfactory cosmetic appearance.[37] Numerous methods of surgical excision and prevention of recurrence have been reported with variable results. Although conjunctival autografts have shown success, they are not feasible to cover large defects created in double-head primary or large recurrent pterygia. Furthermore, concerns have been raised for those who may require future glaucoma-filtering surgeries. In addition, because of graft suturing, this method has the disadvantage of a relatively longer surgery time when compared with the bare sclera technique; also, it carries the risk of complications such as granuloma formation and giant papillary conjunctivitis, as well as significant patient discomfort after surgery.[38] In recent years, a better understanding of the role of limbal stem cells[39] and widespread use of amniotic membrane in pterygium surgery have led to the development of different surgical techniques for this disease.

Surgical Technique

The use of an operating microscope and the standard microsurgical instruments required include 0.12-mm forceps, smooth conjunctival forceps, Wescott scissors, calipers, cautery, microneedle driver (when sutures are used), beaver blade, diamond-dusted burr, and amniotic membrane.

The eye undergoing surgery is prepped and draped in the usual sterile fashion. After anesthesia is applied with either local, subconjunctival, or peribulbar anesthesia, the pterygium is excised with the individual surgeon's preferred technique. The pterygium head is undermined and separated at the limbus and dissected toward the central cornea with Westcott scissors. After excising the head and most of the body, an additional 1 to 2 mm margin of conjunctival tissue is dissected, thus exposing the bare sclera and creating a potential space for the amniotic membrane. Limited cautery is applied as necessary. Scraping the area with a beaver blade and/or diamond-dusted burr on a high-speed drill can remove residual attachments of Tenon's fascia and conjunctiva and is used to smooth the peripheral cornea and limbus. The excised specimen is submitted for pathologic examination to confirm the diagnosis. Next, the amniotic membrane is cut within its surgical packaging to the appropriate size. Amniotic membrane has a basement membrane surface and it is important to leave the basement membrane on top, away from the sclera. With the dry amniotic membrane (AmbioDry 2), the basement membrane side is easily identified when the surgeon can read the letters "IOP" on the graft. In the packaged frozen wet-form, the basement membrane side is on the top surface opposite the cellulose paper on which the amnion is mounted. Surgeons can confirm this by using a cellulose sponge on the surface of the graft; the stromal side is typically stickier than the basement membrane side.[40]

Prior to application of the amniotic membrane, some surgeons like to place MMC in the subconjunctival space to prevent recurrence of pterygium growth. It is important to avoid exposure to bare sclera and to rinse copiously with BSS after removal. If tissue adhesive is not available, the amniotic membrane is secured into position with sutures. More often, however, fibrin glue is used in conjunction with the amniotic membrane. The surgical assistant prepares the 2 components of the Tisseel VH fibrin sealant while the surgeon removes the pterygium. The product may be delivered to the ocular surface in 2 ways to form the fibrin clot. The first technique involves application through the Duploject syringe supplied in the Tisseel VH kit. After combining the 2 components in the Y-connector, 10 drops are wasted before injecting 1 drop under the amniotic membrane. The membrane is then rapidly positioned by smoothing out the membrane over the scleral bed with a smooth instrument. The coagulum (fibrin clot) starts forming in 5 to 7 seconds and achieves 70% of its final tensile strength in 10 minutes with full strength achieved in 2 hours.[4] One can also vary the glue setting times by varying the concentrations and amounts of the 2 components in the mix. In the second technique, one drop of the fibrinogen solution is placed on the scleral bed. Carefully place the amniotic membrane at least a few millimeters beneath the surrounding conjunctival tissue because the fibroblasts that can lead to recurrence reside in this area. Finally, place thrombin on top and around the edges of the amniotic membrane to activate. The amniotic membrane should stay in place for weeks, exerting its antifibrotic and anti-inflammatory effects (Figure 8-3).[41]

At the conclusion of the operation, the speculum is removed and the eye is checked to confirm that the graft is securely in place. An antibiotic-steroid ointment is applied over the ocular surface and the eye is patched and shielded. The patient is instructed to use antibiotics and steroids as per the surgeon's preference.

The above procedure using tissue adhesive rather than sutures may be completed in significantly less time. Moreover, postoperative discomfort is much less than with any type of suture. The eye is generally quieter after fibrin sealant is used than with sutures. This may be explained by the absence of the irritating sutures themselves, the potential anti-inflammatory properties of fibrin glue, or the prevention of peripheral fibroblast migration under the graft.[1] The rate of recurrence of pterygium with this technique appears equal or less than with suture placement.[35]

As with any surgical procedure, there is a learning curve involved with the use of fibrin glue for pterygium surgery. Complications generally arise from using too much product (rarely too little) and not removing excess product out from under the graft. If the glue is not distributed evenly under the graft, the graft may have an edematous appearance in the early postoperative period. Some surgeons do not use thrombin at all in this technique because they feel that the eye's blood supply provides ample native thrombin to facilitate polymerization and graft adhesion. Any part of the underlying sclera not receiving the fibrin glue will lead to poor adherence and retraction of the graft. The surgeon should pay close attention to make sure that the membrane is covering the entire defect.

The combined use of conjunctival autograft and placement of amniotic membrane is usually reserved for high-risk cases that involve large or inflamed pterygia or from recurrences of pterygia. Recurrent pterygium is characterized by hyperproliferation of

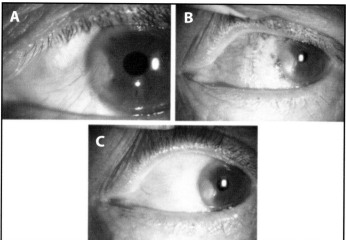

Figure 8-3. De-epithelialized amniotic membrane graft after pterygium excision. (A) External photograph showing pterygium in the right eye before surgery. (B) The appearance 1 week after de-epithelialized amniotic membrane graft. (C) Same eye 8 weeks postoperatively. (Reprinted with permission from Memarzadeh F, Fahd AK, Shamie N, Chuck RS. Comparison of de-epithelialized amniotic membrane transplantation and conjunctival autograft after primary pterygium excision. *Eye.* 2008;22:107-112.)

subconjunctival fibroblasts, resulting in fibrosis with a more accelerated growth rate than primary pterygium. The fibrosis sometimes involves the medial rectus muscle, causing restriction in ocular movement, symblepharon formation, or both. Excision of fibrous tissue with or without conjunctival flap is often insufficient because the underlying disorder—subconjunctival fibrosis—is not treated.[40]

Controversies and Limitations of Amniotic Membrane

The various inhibitory and pro-inflammatory cytokines and other molecules identified in the amniotic membrane have contradictory actions. For instance, IL-6 and IL-8 are pro-inflammatory and, conversely, IL-10 and IL-1ra are anti-inflammatory, yet both are present in the amniotic membrane.[6] Similarly, the presence of various growth factors like epithelial growth factor (EGF) would support epithelial growth and TGF would support wound healing. However, TGF would itself promote scar tissue formation and be contradictory to the "antiadhesive or scar-suppressing action" proposed for the membrane in preventing corneal and conjunctival cicatrization.[14 (p23)] A likely manner in which the amniotic membrane affects its beneficial effect is perhaps as a substrate or basement membrane transplant. It provides a favorable substrate by virtue of its basement membrane for new epithelial cells to migrate on, expand, and adhere. Use of the membrane as a bandage to cover inflamed or exposed areas, due to injury or surgery, not only favorably influences the healing process but also has a dramatic favorable effect on the symptoms of pain or discomfort.[14]

Many differences can exist between amniotic membranes obtained from different donors. Even for the same donor, it is the general practice to obtain numerous pieces of amnion for use in multiple operations. Therefore, some pieces could be from locations closer to the placenta and others distant to it. The thickness of these locations can vary, as can the morphology of the amniotic epithelium. The thickness could affect the integration of the membrane with the ocular surface tissues and perhaps influence the ease with which the membrane comes off at some point after surgery. Age, race, parity, gravidity, and duration of gestation may all contribute to variability of specimens. It is important to keep in mind that membranes used in transplantation are far from standardized across donors and even within the same donor.[14]

Several differences can occur between different membranes depending on whether they are fresh or preserved and, in the case of the latter, on the mode and duration of preservation. Most methods employed in the preservation of the membrane affect it in some manner. The weight of the evidence available supports the notion that the viability of the tissue components of the amniotic membrane is not essential for its biological effectiveness. Until the effect of the different methods of preservation and storage has been evaluated and standardized, success or failure of the membrane should be qualified by the method of preservation employed.

Conclusion

Although not without limitations, AMT has proven success in reducing the recurrence rates in both primary and recurrent pterygia with minimal complications and good cosmetic results. This is accomplished by thoroughly removing the abnormal pterygia tissue; by restoring the matrix in the excision area through the use of the amniotic membrane, which provides a new basement membrane for rapid epithelialization and a stromal matrix for suppressing scarring; and by decreasing inflammation with postoperative use of topical corticosteroids. The main advantage of using amniotic membrane resides in its ability to restore large excised areas (eg, in double-head or large recurrent pterygia), where a conjunctival autograft is not possible. It is also advantageous in cases in which the conjunctiva is already scarred from previous surgery or has to be reserved for a possible glaucoma-filtering surgery. However, further randomized, controlled studies are required to scientifically evaluate the efficacy of the membrane. Perhaps the generation of a synthetic membrane, in which collagen or polymers are used as matrices to incorporate growth factors, cytokines, antimicrobial peptides, and other substances tailored toward specific clinical applications will be possible in the future. This could pave the way to a standardized product with known quantities of desired ingredients in order to generate even more predictable outcomes.

References

1. Hannush S. Pterygium, tissue glue, and the future of wound closure. In: Macsai MS. *Ophthalmic Microsurgical Suturing Techniques.* Heidelberg, Germany: Spring; 2007;135-139.
2. Kucukerdonmez C, Akova Y, Altinors DD. Comparison of conjunctival autograft with amniotic membrane transplantation for pterygium surgery: surgical and cosmetic outcome. *Cornea.* 2007;26:407-413.
3. Trelford JD, Trelford-Sauder M. The amnion in surgery, past and present. *Am J Obstet and Gynecol.* 1979;134:833-845.
4. Schilling B, Yeh J. Transforming growth factor-beta(1), -beta(2), -beta(3) and their type I and II receptors in human term placenta. *Gynecol Obstet Invest.* 2000;50:19-23.
5. Rao CV, Carman FR, Chegini N. Binding sites for epidermal growth factor in human fetal membranes. *J Clin Endocrinol Metab.* 1984;58:1034-1042.
6. Rahman I, Said DG, Maharajan VS, Duah HS. Amniotic membrane in ophthalmology: indications and limitations. *Eye.* 2009;23:1954-1961.
7. Schwan BL. Human amniotic membrane transplantation for the treatment of ocular surface disease. *Northeast Florida Medicine Journal.* Aug-Sep 2002:53(6). Available at: http://www.dcmsonline.org/jax-medicine/2002journals/augsept2002/amniotic.htm. Accessed April 20, 2011.
8. Davis JW. Skin transplantation with a review of 550 cases at the Johns Hopkins Hospital. *Johns Hopkins Med J.* 1910;15:307-396.

9. De Rotth A. Plastic repair of conjunctival defects with fetal membranes. *Arch Ophthalmol.* 1940;23:522-525.

10. Kim JC, Tseng SCG. Transplantation of preserved human amniotic membrane for surface reconstruction in severely damaged rabbit cornea. *Cornea.* 1995;14:473-484.

11. Baradaran-Rafii AR, Aghayan HR, Arjmand B, Javadi MA. Amniotic membrane transplantation. *Iran J Ophthalmic Res.* 2007;2:58-75.

12. Tseng SCG, Li DQ, Ma X. Suppression of transforming growth factor-beta isoforms, TGF-beta receptor type II, and myofibroblast differentiation in cultured human corneal and limbalfibroblasts by amniotic membrane matrix. *J Cell Physiol.* 1999;179:325-35.

13. Shimmura S, Shimazaki J, Ohashi Y, Tsubota K. Antiinflammatory effects of amniotic membrane transplantation in ocular surface disorders. *Cornea.* 2001;20:408-13

14. Dua HS, Maharajan VS, Hopkinson A. Controversies and limitations of amniotic membrane in ophthalmic surgery. In: Reinhard T, Larkin D. *Cornea and External Eye Disease.* Heidelberg, Germany: Springer; 2006:21-23.

15. Figueiredo FC. Amniotic membrane transplantation in ophthalmology. *Royal College of Ophthalmogists Guidelines.* Available at: http://www.mrcophth.com/focus1/Amniotic%20Transplantation.htm. Accessed December 28, 2009.

16. Koizumi NJ, Inatomi TJ, Sotozono CJ, Fullwood NJ, Quantock AJ, Kinoshita S. Growth factor mRNA and protein in preserved human amniotic membrane. *Curr Eye Res.* 2000;20:173-177.

17. Roth I, Corry DB, Locksley RM, Abrams JS, Litton MJ, Fisher SJ. Human placental cytotrophoblasts produce the immunosuppressive cytokine interleukin 10. *J Exp Med.* 1996;184:539-548.

18. Jones CA, Williams KA, Finaly-Jones JJ, Hart PH. Interleukin 4 production by human amnion epithelial cells and regulation of its activity by glycosaminoglycan binding. *Biol Reprod.* 1995;52:839-847.

19. Ueta M, Kweon MN, Sano Y, et al. Immunosuppressive properties of human amniotic membrane for mixed lymphocyte reaction. *Clin Exp Immunol.* 2002;129:464-470.

20. Park CY, Kohanim S, Zhu L, Gehlbach PL, Chuck RS. Immunosuppressive property of dried human amniotic membrane. *Ophthalmic Res.* 2009;41(2):112-113.

21. IOP Opthalmics. Ambio5. 2011. Available at: http://www.iopinc.com/ophthalmic-surgeons/ambio5. Accessed February 5, 2010.

22. Chuck RS, Graff JM, Bryant MR, Sweet PM. Biomechanical characterization of human amniotic membrane preparations for ocular surface reconstruction. *Ophthalmic Res.* 2004;36(6):341-348.

23. Cohen RA, McDonald MB. Fixation of conjunctival autografts with an organic tissue adhesive. *Arch Ophthalmol.* 1993;111:1167-1168.

24. Chan SM, Boisjoly H. Advances in the use of adhesives in ophthalmology. *Curr Opin Ophthalmol.* 2004;15:305-310.

25. Biedner B, Rosenthal G. Conjunctival closure in strabismus surgery: Vicryl versus fibrin glue. *Ophthalmic Surg Lasers.* 1996;27:967.

26. Kaufman HE, Insler MS, Ibrahim-Elzembely HA, Kaufman SC. Human fibrin tissue adhesive for sutureless lamellar keratoplasty and scleral patch adhesion: a pilot study. *Ophthalmology.* 2003;110:2168-2172.

27. O'Sullivan F, Dalton R, Rostron CK. Fibrin glue: an alternative method of wound closure in glaucoma surgery. *J Glaucoma.* 1996;5:367-370.

28. Tisseel [package insert]. Glendale, CA: Baxter Healthcare; 2007.

29. Evicel [package insert]. Somerville, NJ: Johnson & Johnson; 2006.

30. Redl H, Schlag G. Fibrin sealant and its modes of application. In: Schlag G, Redl H, eds. *Fibrin Sealant in Operative Medicine: Volume 2: Ophthalmology-Neurosurgery.* Berlin, Germany: Springer Verlag; 1986:13-25.

31. Schlag G, Ascher PW, Steinkogler FJ, Stammberger H, eds. *Fibrin Sealing in Surgical and Nonsurgical Fields: Volume 5: Neurosurgery, Ophthalmic Surgery, ENT.* Berlin, Germany: Springer Verlag; 1994.

32. Schlag G, Redl H, eds. *Fibrin Sealant in Operative Medicine: Volume 2: Ophthalmology-Neurosurgery.* Berlin, Germany: Springer Verlag; 1986.

33. Srinivasan S, Dollin M, McAllum P, Berger Y, Rootman DS, Slomovic AR. Fibrin glue versus sutures for attaching the conjunctival autograft in pterygium surgery: a prospective observer masked clinical trial. *Br J Ophthalmol.* 2009 93: 215-218.

34. Mangano DT, Tudor IC, Dietzel C. The risk associated with aprotinin in cardiac surgery. *N Engl J Med.* 2006;354,353-365.

35. Por YM, Tan DT. Assessment of fibrin glue in pterygium surgery. *Cornea.* 2010;29:1-4.

36. Koranyi G, Seregard S, Kpp ED. The cut-and-paste method for primary pterygium surgery. *Br J Ophthalmol.* 2004;88:911-914.

37. Solomon A, Pires RTF, Tseng S. Amniotic membrane transplantation after extensive removal of primary and recurrent pterygia. *Ophthalmology.* 2001;108:449-460.

38. Starck T, Kenyon KR, Serrano F. Conjunctival autograft for primary and recurrent pterygia: surgical technique and problem management. *Cornea.* 1991;10:196-202.
39. Sridhar MS, Vemuganti GK, Bansal AK, Rao GN. Impression cytology proven corneal stem cell deficiency in patients after surgeries involving the limbus. *Cornea.* 2001;20:145-148.
40. Hovanesian JA. Three newer methods for treating pterygium: a look at autografting, fibrin adhesives and amnion, a combined approach to improve outcomes. Review of Ophthalmology. Dec 2009. Available at: http://www.revophth.com/content/d/cornea--anterior_segment/i/1209/c/22795/. Accessed April 20, 2011.
41. Shimazaki J, Kosaka K, Shimmura S, Tsubota K. Amniotic membrane transplantation with conjunctival autograft for recurrent pterygium. *Ophthalmology.* 2003;110:119-124.

9

Pterygium Excision With a Conjunctival Autograft and Prophylactic Placement of Subconjunctival Amniotic Membrane Surrounding the Excision Site

John A. Hovanesian, MD and Andrew S. Behesnilian, MD

Rationale

In this chapter, we describe a technique for pterygium excision with conjunctival autograft where pterygium recurrence is prevented by the prophylactic use of subconjunctival amniotic membrane (AM) placed beneath the surrounding, healthy conjunctiva. The addition of this step with AM has, in our experience, provided for quieter healing after surgery, and evidence suggests that it may lead to a lower rate of recurrence than with conjunctival autografting alone. Traditional bare sclera pterygium excision alone or with primary closure carries an unacceptably high rate of recurrence (up to 80%) and has largely been abandoned.[1]

Medicinal adjuncts such as mitomycin-C (MMC) may reduce the rate of recurrence but, especially in high doses, is significantly associated with persistent epithelial defects of both cornea and sclera, scleral necrosis, infectious scleritis, and even endophthalmitis and perforation.[2]

For the treatment of pterygium, many cornea specialists currently prefer surgical excision with use of a conjunctival autograft (CA). This technique, which is attributed to Dr. Ken Kenyon, involves filling the void of the excised pterygium with a graft of the patient's adjacent conjunctiva. Recurrences with this technique occur at a rate of up to 10%.[1]

An alternative to CA is to fill the void of the excision site with AM. AM is derived from human placental tissue and has been used regularly in ocular surface surgery since 1940 because of its well known anti-inflammatory and antiscarring effects. AM is thought to prevent fibrosis by inhibiting cytokine expression by fibroblasts and IL-1 by

Hovanesian JA. *Pterygium: Techniques and Technologies for Surgical Success* (pp 101-110)
© 2012 Taylor & Francis Group

epithelial cells, as well as by suppressing fibroblast differentiation and proliferation.[3] AM also has been successfully used in procedures for neurotrophic corneal ulcers, chemical or thermal burns,[4] and as a tectonic patch.[5] It is available commercially under the same Food and Drug Administration (FDA) regulation that governs eye bank tissue. When used in place of a CA, AM has been successful in reducing the recurrence of pterygia compared to bare sclera excision; however, recurrence rates are still comparable to CA, at about 10%.[6]

It has been commonly observed that pterygium recurrences arise from the subconjunctival Tenon's fascia surrounding the excision site. Neither CA nor surface placement of AM actively address this source tissue. For this reason, we have used AM in a simple adjunctive procedure that can be performed with pterygium excision and CA. In this procedure, a small strip of amniotic membrane is placed in the subconjunctival space surrounding the pterygium excision before placement of a CA.[7]

The technique described in this chapter of "CA with prophylactic placement of subconjunctival AM" (CA/AM) would allow the antifibrotic and anti-inflammatory effects of AM to be in contact with the location from which pterygium recurrence arises. In placing the amnion under the conjunctival surface, it is protected from the frictional forces of blinking and the melting effects of constant tear turnover and is likely to remain present for much longer than the 2 to 3 weeks normally associated with a surface AM graft. In this subconjunctival location, the AM is thought to function as a biologic depot of antifibrotic and anti-inflammatory material that prevents pterygium recurrence.

In this technique, fibrin tissue adhesive is used to secure both the CA and AM. Fibrin adhesive has been used for over 25 years for the repair of splenic and liver rupture and as an adjunct in cardiac surgery. It has been used extensively in place of sutures in pterygium surgery because it allows more comfortable healing after surgery with less inflammation.[8] In this application, the thrombin component of fibrin adhesive is diluted 1:9 with balanced salt solution (BSS). This dilution does not weaken the adhesive's tensile strength but significantly slows the polymerization time, giving the surgeon additional time to manipulate tissues before the adhesive "sets."[9]

Results

Performing a rigorous prospective controlled study comparing any one pterygium technique to another would require a large number of subjects because of the fairly low (about 1% in our experience) incidence of recurrence with established procedures. The high individual variability of pterygium patients also would complicate the analysis. Risk factors that contribute to recurrence such as young age, male gender, dark-skin, pterygium size, degree of preoperative inflammation, presence of dry eye, and prior recurrence would need to be equalized between treatment and control groups. To achieve statistical power, such a study would require more patients than can be recruited in a reasonable time, even by multiple centers.

A retrospective analysis of 80 patients who underwent the CA/AM procedure revealed no recurrences in a 13-month follow-up period. Postoperatively, all conjunctival and AM grafts remained viable and in place. One eye developed a pyogenic granuloma at the nasal edge of its autograft. This did not require further surgical intervention and resolved over 6 weeks with topical steroid treatment.[10]

Further anecdotal evidence exists supporting the value of the combined use of CA and AM. In one case, a 52-year-old patient with bilateral, asymmetrical pterygia

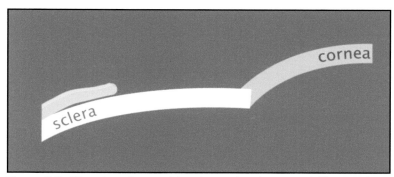

Figure 9-1. After pterygium excision, bare sclera is exposed. Note conjunctiva is shown in pink, with a yellow line on its epithelial side. (Reprinted with permission of John A. Hovanesian, MD.)

underwent a different procedure in each eye. The right eye was not inflamed but had a 2-mm nasal pterygium, while the left eye had a heavily vascularized, inflamed pterygium extending 3 mm onto the nasal cornea. No other discernible difference existed between the eyes. On the left eye, the patient had pterygium excision with a CA and prophylactic placement of subconjunctival AM. The postoperative course was uneventful. One year later, the patient requested surgery on his right eye. At this time, the left eye had a well-healed graft. Because the right eye's pterygium was less aggressive, the patient had a CA alone. The procedure was performed by the same surgeon (Dr. John A. Hovanesian) and initial postoperative course was uneventful. However, unlike the left eye, which had a more inflamed and larger pterygium, the right eye unexpectedly developed a recurrence 2 months after surgery.

Surgical Technique

The pterygium is excised along with an additional 1-mm margin of conjunctival tissue, exposing the bare sclera (Figure 9-1). Next, blunt Westcott scissors are used to create a potential space beneath the conjunctiva surrounding the excision site, tunneling about 5 mm into this tissue on all 3 sides. This potential space should be superficial to most of Tenon's fascia, the medial rectus muscle, and tendon. Minimal cautery is used to establish hemostasis. Next, a thin CA similar in size to the conjunctival defect that was created after pterygium excision is prepared from the superior bulbar conjunctiva of the same eye. At this point, the graft is left attached at the limbus superiorly (Figure 9-2), such that it is not misplaced during the subsequent surgical steps.

Amniotic Membrane Preparation

In this procedure it is possible to use either cryopreserved or freeze-dried human AM. However, clinical experience has shown that thinner (freeze-dried) AM material is easier to place in the subconjunctival space. The most suitable freeze-dried preparation we have found is AmbioDry 2 (IOP Ophthalmics, Costa Mesa, CA), with a dry thickness of about 35 µm. In its dry form, this material is removed from the outer packaging but is left in its inner packaging. The AM is then cut through the packaging into a C-shaped graft that is large enough to surround the conjunctival defect (Figure 9-3). If the wet form of AM is used (Amniograft, BioTissue, Inc, Miami, FL), it is similarly cut into a C-shaped graft on the supplied paper.

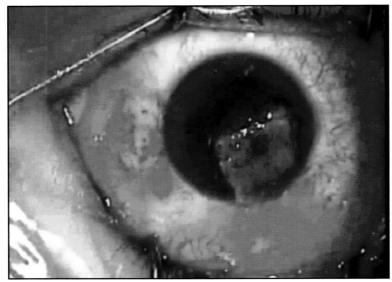

Figure 9-2. The pterygium has been excised and the autograft prepared and reflected onto the cornea at the superior limbus. (Reprinted with permission of John A. Hovanesian, MD.)

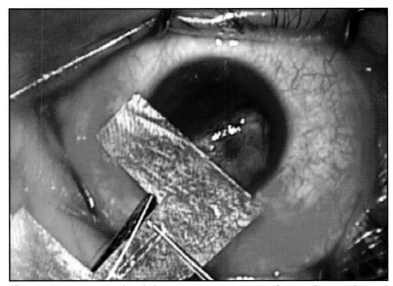

Figure 9-3. Freeze-dried human amniotic membrane is cut into a C-shaped graft. (Reprinted with permission of John A. Hovanesian, MD.)

Fibrin Adhesive Preparation

Fibrin tissue adhesive (Tisseel [Baxter Healthcare Corp, Deerfield, IL] or Evicel [Ethicon, Inc, Somerville, NJ]) is prepared according to the manufacturer's instructions, but the components are not transferred to the supplied double-barrel syringe. These vials are held by a circulating nurse, and the top of each is wiped with rubbing alcohol to minimize contamination during transfer. The gloved scrub nurse then draws approximately 0.1 cc of each into 2 separate, sterile 1-cc syringes through a sterile 18-gauge needle. Air entry into these syringes is minimized. Next, 0.9 cc of BSS is

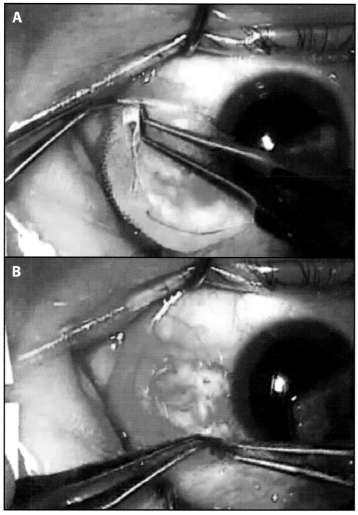

Figure 9-4. The amnionic membrane is tucked into the subconjunctival space surrounding the site of pterygium excision to provide its antifibrotic effects to Tenon's fascia, from which pterygium recurrence might arise. (Reprinted with permission of John A. Hovanesian, MD.)

added into the thrombin-filled syringe, and the syringe is inverted several times to facilitate mixing. The adhesive components are now ready for use.

Amniotic Membrane Application

The cut-edge of the conjunctiva is lifted using 0.12 forceps, and a Paton spatula (Katena Eye Instruments, Denville, NJ) containing a small droplet of fibrinogen is introduced. The fibrinogen is applied to the undersurface of the conjunctiva that was tented. This fibrinogen will help keep the AM in place upon its introduction into this surgically-created potential space in the subconjunctival region. Thrombin is not applied at this time. Next, a few drops of sterile BSS are placed on the bare sclera that will allow for the subsequent hydration of the freeze-dried AM and facilitate its ability to slide onto the ocular surface. This step is not necessary if the wet form of AM is used. The AM graft is removed from its packaging and placed on the bare sclera. Using nontoothed, smooth forceps, the AM is then gently grasped and brought into the subconjunctival space (Figure 9-4). The membrane is evenly distributed in this space. Some AM folds may remain, which usually have no postoperative deleterious effects on

Figure 9-5. (A) The figure shows the location of the amniotic membrane in red around the eventual location of the conjunctival autograft. (B) Amniotic membrane (red) does not cover the bare sclera defect. (Reprinted with permission of John A. Hovanesian, MD.)

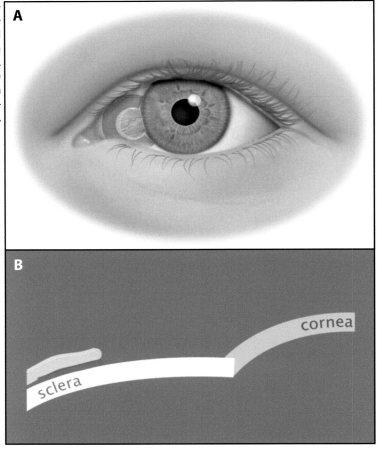

the overall outcome of this surgical procedure. The goal is to create a subconjunctival AM "beltway" that surrounds the area of the bare sclera, not to cover the bare sclera (Figure 9-5). After placing the AM in the subconjunctival space, the edges of the overlying conjunctiva are lifted and advanced toward the limbus to cover any remnants of AM transplantation that are exposed. The presence of the fibrinogen, mixed with small amounts of thrombin in the patient's own blood, will allow these edges to stay in place, covering all of the AM transplantation.

Application of Conjunctival Autograft

The CA, which remains attached to the superior limbus, is now reflected onto the cornea (epithelium to epithelium) and cut free from the superior limbus with scissors (Figure 9-6). The surgeon slides this graft across the cornea, orienting its limbal side to the limbus where the pterygium was excised (Figure 9-7). A small droplet from the diluted thrombin syringe is applied to the bare sclera (Figure 9-8), and a small droplet from the fibrinogen syringe is applied to the underside of the graft. The graft is then grasped with 2 MacPherson forceps and flipped onto the bare sclera. This allows the 2 adhesive components to mix, and the surgeon has about 30 seconds to manipulate and orient the graft appropriately, such that the edges of the graft are approximated with the cut edges of the surrounding conjunctiva and the corneal margin is aligned with the limbus (Figure 9-9).

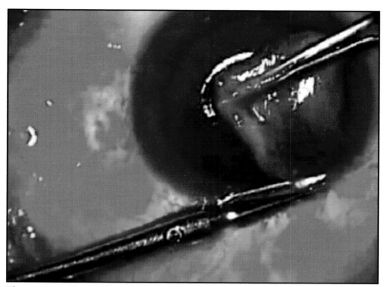

Figure 9-6. From the superior limbus, the conjunctival autograft is cut free. (Reprinted with permission of John A. Hovanesian, MD.)

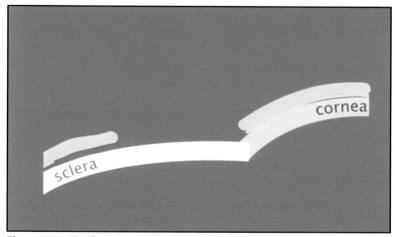

Figure 9-7. The free conjunctival autograft is inverted on the cornea (note yellow epithelial surface of graft shown against the corneal epithelium) and oriented limbus-to-limbus adjacent to the excision site. (Reprinted with permission of John A. Hovanesian, MD.)

Surgical Pearls

- Conservative use of cautery avoids postoperative pain and is usually sufficient as the fibrin adhesive provides additional hemostasis.
- Dilution of 1 part thrombin with 9 parts BSS slows the polymerization process with fibrin adhesive and allows more time to manipulate the graft.
- Harvesting a thin CA is best accomplished by making a small opening in the conjunctiva distal to the limbus and then lifting the cut edge of the conjunctiva (with minimal Tenon's membrane) using toothed forceps. Blunt Westcott scissors can

Figure 9-8. Thrombin (shown in black) diluted with BSS is placed on the excision site, and fibrinogen (shown in blue) is placed on the stromal side of the autograft. (Reprinted with permission of John A. Hovanesian, MD.)

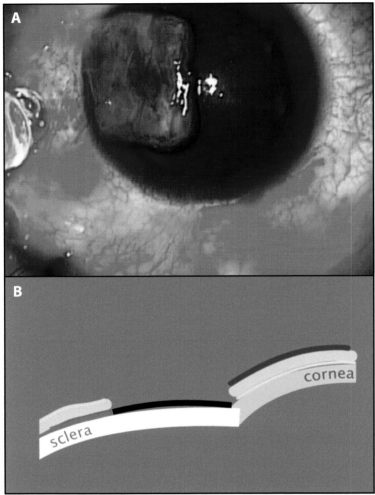

be inserted parallel to the conjunctival surface and then opened in the plane just below the conjunctiva to separate it away from the underlying tissues, namely most of Tenon's membrane.

- The CA should match the size of the conjunctival opening after pterygium excision and should not be significantly oversized or contain excessive Tenon's membrane in order to avoid any significant tissue swelling after surgery.

- Once the CA is in place covering the bare sclera with its edge properly approximated (as described above) and the 2 components of the fibrin glue begin to mix, the surgeon should avoid unnecessary touching of the graft or surrounding conjunctiva as this will usually weaken the "bonds" of the fibrin adhesive and may result in suboptimal attachment of the CA.

- During the postoperative follow-up period, a small gap at the nasal edge of the graft may occasionally occur. This does not increase the risk of recurrence of the pterygium.

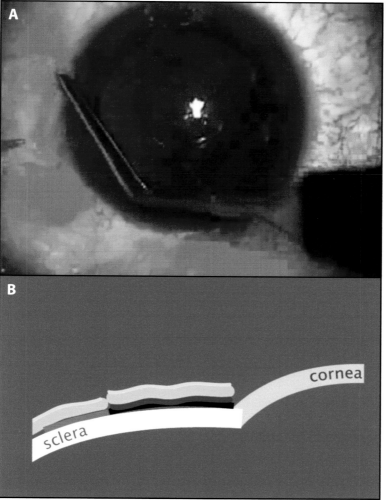

Figure 9-9. The conjunctival autograft is inverted, mixing the adhesive components, and smoothed to approximate the edges of conjunctiva. (Reprinted with permission of John A. Hovanesian, MD.)

Postoperative Follow-Up/Drug Regimen

A topical fluoroquinolone antibiotic is applied 4 times a day (QID) for 1 week after surgery. Prednisolone acetate 1% is started QID and tapered over 4 more weeks. Additionally, we prescribe a topical nonsteroidal anti-inflammatory drug to manage pain for the first few days after surgery.

Conclusion

The CA/AM technique described in this chapter has been used with success as an adjunct to simple conjunctival autografting in pterygium cases with a higher risk of recurrence. This includes large, inflamed, or recurrent pterygia. It takes advantage of AM's antifibrotic effects and positions them directly in contact with the subconjunctival Tenon's fascia that is thought to be the source of recurrence. This avoids the need for extensive dissection of Tenon's with attendant risks of scarring and muscle restriction.

Although it can be combined with MMC or other antimetabolites, it is generally not necessary to expose the patient to the risks of these materials. In the expanding array of options for pterygium surgeons, we have found that this technique offers a fairly simple prophylactic adjunct that improves upon results with current techniques.

References

1. Kenyon KR, Wagoner MD, Hettinger ME. Conjunctival autograft transplantation for advanced and recurrent pterygium. *Ophthalmology.* 1985;92:1461-1470.
2. Rubinfeld RS, Pfister RR, Stein RM, et al. Serious complications of topical mitomycin-C after pterygium surgery. *Ophthalmology.* 1992;99:1647-1654.
3. Choi TH, Tseng SC. In vivo and in vitro demonstration of epithelial cell-induced myofibroblast differentiation of keratocytes and an inhibitory effect by amniotic membrane. *Cornea.* 2001;20:197-204.
4. Shimazaki J, Yang HY, Tsubota K. Amniotic membrane transplantation for ocular surface reconstruction in patients with chemical and thermal burns. *Ophthalmology.* 1997;104(12):2068-2076.
5. Azuara-Blanco A, Pillai CT, Dua HS. Amniotic membrane transplantation for ocular surface reconstruction. *Br J Ophthalmol.* 1999;83(4):399-402.
6. Memarzadeh F, Fahd AK, Shamie N, Chuck RS. Comparison of de-epithelialized amniotic membrane transplantation and conjunctival autograft after primary pterygium excision. *Eye (Lond).* 2008;22(1):107-112.
7. Hovanesian JA, Behesnilian A. Results of pterygium excision using amniotic membrane beneath the healthy conjunctiva surrounding a conjunctival autograft. Poster presented at: Annual Meeting of the American Society of Cataract and Refractive Surgery; 2008; Chicago, IL.
8. Koranyi G, Seregard S, Kopp ED. Cut and paste: a no suture, small incision approach to pterygium surgery. *Br J Ophthalmol.* 2004;88(7):911-914.
9. Hovanesian JA. Does "slow set" dilution of fibrin tissue adhesive reduce its strength in ocular surgery? Paper presented at: American Society of Cataract and Refractive Surgery Symposium; 2007; San Diego, CA.
10. Hovanesian JA. Amnionic membrane as an antifibrotic implant in the subconjunctival space surrounding a conjunctival autograft in pterygium surgery. Poster presented at: American Academy of Ophthalmology Meeting; 2008; Atlanta, GA.

10

Pterygium
Postoperative Management and Complications

Dhivya Ashok Kumar, MD and Amar Agarwal, MS, FRCS, FRCOphth

Pterygium is a subconjunctival fibrotic and degenerative condition usually treated with surgical removal. The methods of pterygium surgery vary from the simplest bare sclera excision to sophisticated keratoplasty. The treatment of pterygium does not end with mechanical removal of the mass lesion alone. Moreover, proper postoperative medications, regular follow-up, and postoperative complications management completes the overall treatment protocol. Postoperative complications are not uncommon in pterygium excision. It can be due to the surgical technique, adjuvants used like antimetabolites, sutures, medications, or the disease, per se. Recurrence and residual scarring is commonly experienced in our clinical practice. This can be seen in the early or late postoperative period. Vision-threatening complications like corneal perforation, melting, and postoperative infections, although rare, are also reported.

Postoperative Management

The routine medications include topical antibiotics, lubricants, and analgesics in the immediate postoperative period.

Immediate Postoperative Care

All patients operated for pterygium should be seen at the slit lamp within 2 to 3 days of surgery. Visual acuity, intraocular pressure, and corneal clarity should be recorded. The position of the graft (amniotic membrane graft [AMG] or conjunctival autograft) and bleeding sites, if noted, should be documented. The patient should be advised not to squeeze or rub the eyes in the immediate postoperative period and should also be prescribed topical medications.

Hovanesian JA. *Pterygium: Techniques and Technologies for Surgical Success (pp 111-120)*
© 2012 Taylor & Francis Group

Prophylactic Antibiotics

Third-generation fluoroquinolones (0.3% gatifloxacin or 0.5% moxifloxacin) are commonly used for postoperative prophylaxis. Drugs in drop formulations are more compliant than ointments. The addition of aminoglycosides (tobramycin) is optional. Commonly, a 4 times daily dose is preferred. Some surgeons use antibiotic steroid combinations. Topical prednisolone acetate 1% and tobramycin 0.3% combination (TobraDex) can be used 4 times daily after surgery and tapered off.

The end point of topical corticosteroids usage is determined based on sufficient disappearance of inflammation, as determined by slit-lamp findings.

Lubricants

Pterygium patients can have associated dry eye changes. There have been reports[1,2] showing the improvement in tear film functions after pterygium excision. Therefore, we recommend postoperative lubricants in the immediate postoperative period. Carboxymethyl cellulose (0.5% or 1%) can be used 4 times daily for 2 weeks. Avoidance of dry air exposure and excessive outdoor work are recommended in high-risk patients.

Analgesics

As in any surgical procedure, postoperative pain can be alleviated with simple analgesics and anti-inflammatory agents. Topical anti-inflammatory (nonsteroidal anti-inflammatory drug [NSAID]) drops like bromfenac are usually preferred; however, patients with a low pain threshold may require oral anti-inflammatory agents as well.

Topical Mitomycin-C

Topical mitomycin-C (MMC) is given only for selected patients with multiple recurrences or severe fibrosis. A topical 0.02% dose can be used. Patients with topical MMC application should be followed up with regularly because of its known corneal and ocular surface side effects, which will be explained in the complications of MMC section on page 119.

Protective Glasses

Since dryness and exposure have been associated with pterygium, postoperative ultraviolet (UV) protection glasses can be advised in specific patients.

Complications After Pterygium Excision

Immediate Complications

- Excessive bleeding due to reactionary hemorrhage can be noted in the immediate postoperative period. A pressure bandage usually controls this. Patients with systemic hypertension should continue their antihypertensive medications.

- Conjunctival chemosis can be seen in few patients and will resolve spontaneously.

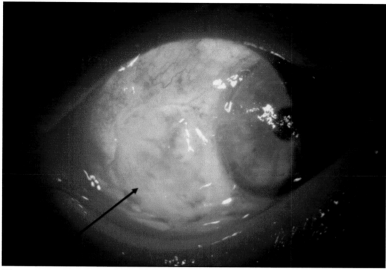

Figure 10-1. Day 1 postoperative after pterygium excision with conjunctival autograft graft. Graft edema (arrow) seen.

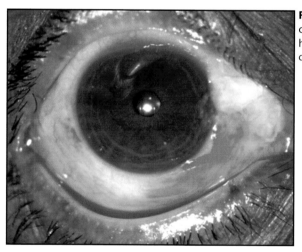

Figure 10-2. Postoperative picture after conjunctival autograft showing subgraft-hemorrhage with minimal corneal epithelial defect.

- Graft edema (Figure 10-1) may be seen and will resolve with topical treatment.
- Hematoma below the graft may occur due to persistent bleeding because of improper hemostasis. In this case, the graft is examined under the microscope and the hematoma evacuated under a block.
- Localized epithelial defect is seen in almost all patients on postoperative day 1 (Figure 10-2). This will heal within 24 hours.
- Corneal scar, either a macular or nebular opacity depending upon the depth of corneal involvement, may be observed from the immediate postoperative period (Figure 10-3). Excess scar or deep opacity may require lamellar keratoplasty at a later time.

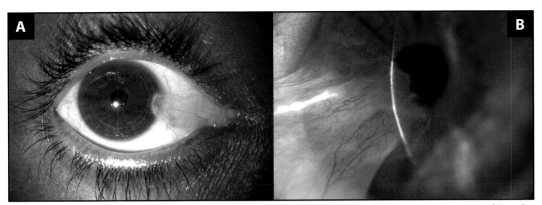

Figure 10-3. (A) Early pterygium with minimal corneal involvement. (B) Thick pterygium encroaching the cornea with scarring.

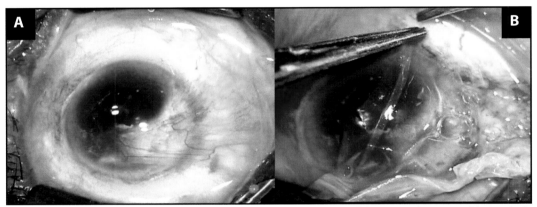

Figure 10-4. (A) A large recurrent pterygium with deeper corneal layer involvement. (B) Amniotic membrane graft is placed after pterygium excision.

Late Complications

Recurrence

One of the major limitations of pterygium excision is the high rate of postoperative recurrence. The recurrence time ranges from months to years. Increased fibroblastic activity is a well-established finding in recurrent pterygia. Recurrent pterygium is more difficult to treat than primary pterygium because it is often accompanied by increased conjunctival inflammation and accelerated corneal involvement (Figure 10-4A). Partial limbal stem cell deficiency and coexisting inflammation might be one of the etiologies for recurrent pterygia. Bare sclera surgery has the highest relapse rate after pterygium removal.[3] The recurrence rate was 10.9% (in primary pterygium), 37.5% (recurrent pterygium), and 14.8% (all pterygium) after pterygium excision with amniotic membrane graft in a study by Prabhasawat et al.[4] Conjunctival autograft showed a recurrence of 2.6% (in primary pterygium), 9.1% (recurrent pterygium), and 4.9% (all pterygium), which was far less than other methods.

Treatment

Preoperative, intraoperative, and postoperative use of antimetabolites, namely MMC, reduces the risk of recurrence.[5-7] Lee et al has reported that MMC effects are stronger in recurrent pterygium than with primary cells.[8] Conjunctival autograft with pterygium excision is known to show less recurrence and is the first choice of surgical treatment.[4,9] Limbal stem cell transplantation can improve ocular surface in eyes with recurrent pterygium with limbal stem cell deficiency. Amniotic membrane is a good alternate choice to reduce recurrence in advanced cases with bilateral heads (Figure 10-4B).[9] The postoperative instillation of MMC 0.02% (0.2 mg/mL) eye drops twice daily for 5 days following excision of primary pterygium has been used to reduce recurrence.[10] Topical bevacizumab (5 mg/mL) twice a day has been shown to delay the recurrence in impending recurrent pterygia.[11] Single-dose beta irradiation after bare sclera surgery in the postoperative period is a simple, effective, and safe treatment that reduces the risk of primary pterygium recurrence. A Strontium (Sr)-90 eye applicator is used to deliver 2500 cGy to the sclera surface at a dose rate of between 200 and 250 cGy/min.[12]

Complications of Mitomycin-C

Topical

MMC is an antimetabolite agent produced by a strain of *Streptomyces caespitosus*. It inhibits synthesis of DNA, RNA, and proteins. This drug is referred to as *radio-mimetic* because its action mimics that of ionizing radiation. Topical 0.02% eye drops have been known to cause ocular complications such as superficial punctate keratitis, avascularized sclera, and pyogenic granuloma. Ocular discomfort and lacrimation are some of the common complaints.[10] The use of MMC 0.5 mg/mL has also been used after pterygium excision and beta irradiation, which lead to complications such as scleromalacia, scleral ulcer, and cataract.[13]

Intraoperative Mitomycin-C

Scleral dellen is an early postoperative complication of bare sclera technique with MMC owing to delayed conjunctival wound closure.[14] Treated sclera may become white or "porcelainized" due to destroyed vessels and remain so forever. It has been reported that it is due to the drug's effect on multipotential cells and the rapidly proliferating cells of vascular endothelium.[15] Complications including temporary and prolonged discomfort, tearing, hyperemia, subconjunctival hemorrhage, wound dehiscence, and pigment accumulation with single dose of intraoperative MMC were also noted by Anduze and Burnett.[16] Therefore, it is recommended that only high-risk pterygia receive MMC. Conjunctiva should cover the sclera up to the limbus and thereby prevent migration of MMC. They concluded that a single dose of 0.5 mg/mL subconjunctivally gives the same results as multiple drops, but with far less morbidity. In our experience, short-term low-dose (0.02%) topical postoperative MMC has not caused any vision-threatening complications after pterygium surgery when used in specific patients.

Suture-Related Inflammation

Suture-related inflammation is commonly seen with polyglactin sutures. Proper intraoperative aseptic precautions and postoperative antibiotic applications can reduce it. Some surgeons prefer to use monofilament nylon for suturing the autograft due to increased inflammation with Vicryl sutures (Ethicon Inc, Somerville, NJ). This has recently reduced with the introduction of fibrin glue application for conjunctival autograft (Figure 10-5) and amniotic membrane adhesion.

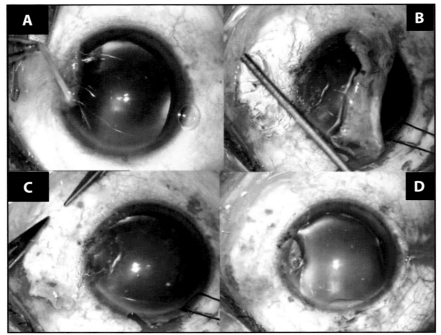

Figure 10-5. Pterygium excision with conjunctival autograft and fibrin glue application. (A) Pterygium excised. (B) Fibrin glue applied in the underlying scleral bed. (C) Conjunctival autograft placed over the glue. (D) Graft well apposed on table.

Tenon's Cyst

This can occur in eyes in which the Tenon's layer was exposed. Excision of the cyst with complete closure is recommended. Improper conjunctival autograft separation, in which the conjunctiva is harvested with thick Tenon's layer, may be a risk factor for this complication.

Diplopia and Strabismus

Scarring and excessive fibrosis in the region of pterygium or in the conjunctiva can lead to restriction of extra ocular movements and diplopia. Patients who have a tendency toward keloid formation and hypertrophic scar are at a high risk of developing such complications. Excess scarring can occasionally cause restrictive strabismus. In such cases, scar exploration and release of fibrosis is usually performed.

Scleral Complications

Scleral ulceration was observed in 51 eyes after pterygium excision with bare sclera surgery on long-term follow-up by Tarr and Constable.[17] *Pseudomonas* endophthalmitis was reported in 4 patients with scleral ulceration after pterygium excision. Tarr and Constable observed that beta irradiation to prevent recurrence of pterygia is a significant cause of iatrogenic ocular disease. Excessive intraoperative cautery to the scleral bed should be avoided. Overuse of antimetabolites can also lead to scleral complications. Necrotizing scleritis has been reported after conjunctival autograft.[18] Scleral thinning with perforation can also occur (Figure 10-6). A complete postoperative clinical evaluation for collagen vascular diseases is recommended in these cases. Nevertheless, prompt diagnosis, systemic immunosuppressant, and early surgical closure with scleral patch graft (Figure 10-7) might prevent further complications.

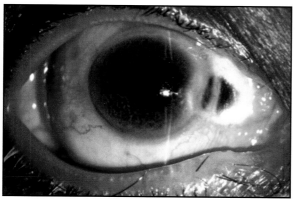

Figure 10-6. Acute scleral thinning with uveal show after pterygium removal.

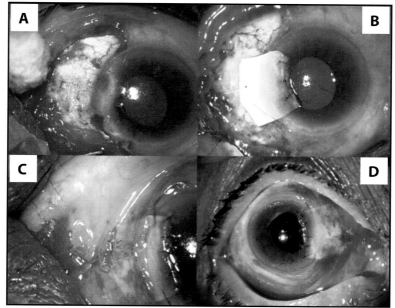

Figure 10-7. Management of complication of scleral thinning after pterygium surgery. (A) Thinned scleral bed area exposed. (B) Donor scleral patch graft placed and sutured to the scleral bed and cornea. (C) Conjunctiva well apposed. (D) Day 1 postoperative picture showing good graft apposition.

Corneal Perforation

Pterygium excision can lead to corneal thinning. We have seen corneal perforation in 2 eyes with a history of excessive straining after pterygium excision. One patient had intraoperative MMC and the other patient had excessive scarring. Corneal patch graft was performed for both patients. Corneoscleral perforation with iris prolapse was also reported by Dadeya and Fatima after intraoperative MMC.[19]

Graft Reversal

Conjunctival autograft can turn from the scleral bed with one end of the graft hanging. This can happen when the conjunctiva has not been stuck properly with fibrin glue or if the sutures are loose. The possible reasons for poor adhesion are due to improper application of tissue glue or sutures. Patients should be taken to the operation theater again and graft repositioning performed.

Lens Changes

Radiation-induced cataract occurred in 3 (4.7%) out of 63 eyes of 57 patients in a study by Tarr and Constable.[17] Sectorial lens opacities with normal visual acuity was seen in 19 eyes in their follow-up.

Miscellaneous

Ptosis, symblepharon, and iris atrophy were also seen after pterygium excision with irradiation. Ptosis will frequently resolve spontaneously over several months. If symptomatic, the symblepharon release can be performed and the patient prescribed topical lubricants.

Conclusion

Postoperative management can invariably be improved by regular follow-up and early detection of complications after pterygium surgery. Amniotic membrane grafting or conjunctival autograft is useful in minimizing the risk of recurrence. Suture-related inflammation is controlled with the recent introduction of sutureless techniques using tissue glue.

References

1. Li M, Zhang M, Lin Y, et al. Tear function and goblet cell density after pterygium excision. *Eye.* 2007;21:224-228.
2. Ishioka M, Shimmura S, Yagi Y, Tsubota K. Pterygium and dry eye. *Ophthalmologica.* 2001;215(3):209-211.
3. Alpay A, Uğurbaş SH, Erdoğan B. Comparing techniques for pterygium surgery. *Clin Ophthalmol.* 2009;3:69-74.
4. Prabhasawat P, Barton K, Burkett G, Tseng SC. Comparison of conjunctival autografts, amniotic membrane grafts, and primary closure for pterygium excision. *Ophthalmology.* 1997;104(6):974-985.
5. Donnenfeld ED, Perry HD, Fromer S, Doshi S, Solomon R, Biser S. Subconjunctival mitomycin C as adjunctive therapy before pterygium excision. *Ophthalmology.* 2003;110:1012-1016.
6. Frucht-Pery J, Siganos CS, Ilsar M. Intraoperative application of topical mitomycin C for pterygium surgery. *Ophthalmology.* 1996;103:674-677.
7. Frucht-Pery J, Ilsar M. The use of low-dose mitomycin C for prevention of recurrent pterygium. *Ophthalmology.* 1994;101:759-762.
8. Lee JS, Oum BS, Lee SH. Mitomycin C influence on inhibition of cellular proliferation and subsequent synthesis of type I collagen and laminin in primary and recurrent pterygia. *Ophthalmic Res.* 2001;33:140-146.
9. Luanratanakorn P, Ratanapakorn T, Suwan-Apichon O, Chuck RS. Randomised controlled study of conjunctival autograft versus amniotic membrane graft in pterygium excision. *Br J Ophthalmol.* 2006;90(12):1476-1480.
10. Rachmiel R, Leiba H, Levartovsky S. Results of treatment with topical mitomycin C 0.02% following excision of primary pterygium. *Br J Ophthalmol.* 1995;79(3):233-236.
11. Fallah MR, Khosravi K, Hashemian MN, Beheshtnezhad AH, Rajabi MT, Gohari M. Efficacy of topical bevacizumab for inhibiting growth of impending recurrent pterygium. *Curr Eye Res.* 2010;35(1):17-22.
12. Jürgenliemk-Schulz IM, Hartman LJ, Roesink JM, et al. Prevention of pterygium recurrence by postoperative single-dose beta-irradiation: a prospective randomized clinical double-blind trial. *Int J Radiat Oncol Biol Phys.* 2004;59(4):1138-1147.
13. Saifuddin S, el Zawawi A. Scleral changes due to mitomycin C after pterygium excision: a report of two cases. *Indian J Ophthalmol.* 1995;43(2):75-76.

14. Tsai YY, Lin JM, Shy JD. Acute scleral thinning after pterygium excision with intraoperative mitomycin C: a case report of scleral dellen after bare sclera technique and review of the literature. *Cornea.* 2002;21(2):227-229.

15. Rubinfeld RS, Pfister PR, Stein RM, et al. Severe complications of topical mitomycin-C after pterygium surgery. *Ophthalmology.* 1992;99:1647-1654.

16. Anduze AL, Burnett JM. Indications for and complications of mitomycin-C in pterygium surgery. *Ophthalmic Surg Lasers.* 1996;27(8):667-673.

17. Tarr KH, Constable IJ. Late complications of pterygium treatment. *Br J Ophthalmol.* 1980;64:496-505.

18. Jain V, Shome D, Natarajan S, Narverkar R. Surgically induced necrotizing scleritis after pterygium surgery with conjunctival autograft. *Cornea.* 2008;27(6):720-721.

19. Dadeya S, Fatima S. Comeoscleral perforation after pterygium excision and intraoperative mitomycin C. *Ophthalmic Surg Lasers Imaging.* 2003;34(2):146-148.

11

Management of
Recurrent Pterygium

Jay C. Bradley, MD

Pterygia are a complicated ocular surface disease that can be difficult to treat effectively. Due to the high prevalence of pterygia, especially in certain populations, proper management is crucial to minimize the risk of recurrences and additional visual defects. Advanced or recurrent pterygia can lead to vision loss due to loss of corneal transparency within the visual axis and irregular corneal astigmatism due to localized flattening (Figure 11-1).[1]

Depending on the technique used for pterygium excision, the recurrence rate varies significantly.[2-4] Bare scleral techniques have largely been abandoned due to unacceptably high rates of recurrence. Although the debate regarding the optimal technique continues, many surgeons currently employ graft closure and/or other adjunctive agents to decrease the risk of recurrent disease, especially in at-risk patients. Risk factors for recurrence include history of prior recurrence, young age, present or past residence in low latitudes or desert climate, outdoor occupation, large pterygium size, increased pterygium thickness or fleshiness, and frequent inflammatory episodes.[1] Postoperative alterations in peripheral corneal topography, persistent wetting defects, and chronic irritation and inflammation after surgery may also increase the likelihood of pterygium recurrence. Although the risk of recurrences with the advancement of surgical techniques and adjunctive therapies has decreased significantly, recurrences continue to be a significant problem for surgeons.

Persistent vascularity and inflammation is often the first clinical sign of recurrence. If untreated, this finding is followed by centripetal movement of this vascularity in the direction of the limbus (Figure 11-2). As this moves toward the limbus, the tissue thickens, clinically resembling the preoperative appearance of the pterygium tissue (Figure 11-3). The recurrent pterygium continues toward the limbus and then finally onto the corneal surface (Figure 11-4). Medical therapies may have some efficacy in the treatment of early recurrences, but for later conjunctival or actual corneal recurrences, they are of questionable utility. Repeat surgical intervention is often required for more advanced recurrences (Figure 11-5). Recurrent pterygia should be considered a different clinical entity as compared to primary pterygia.

Hovanesian JA. *Pterygium: Techniques and Technologies for Surgical Success* (pp 121-134)

Figure 11-1. Recurrent pterygium extending near the visual axis, inducing with-the-rule astigmatism, and causing reduced visual acuity.

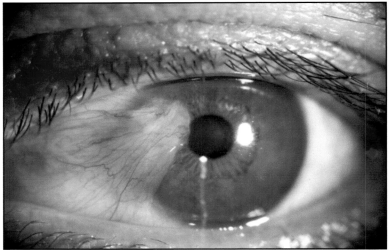

Figure 11-2. Early conjunctival recurrence after pterygium excision using a conjunctival autograft.

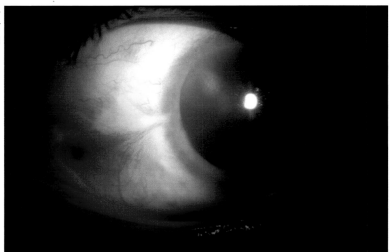

Figure 11-3. Aggressive conjunctival recurrence after pterygium excision using a conjunctival autograft.

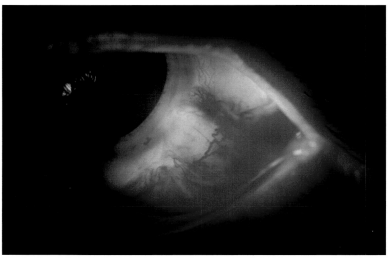

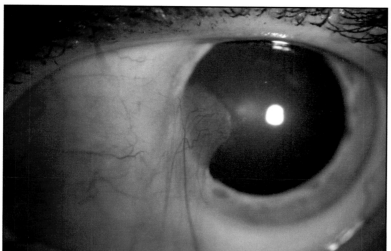

Figure 11-4. Recurrent pterygium after prior excision with conjunctival autograft.

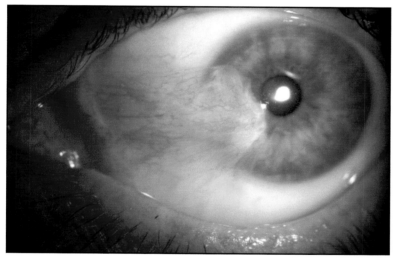

Figure 11-5. Advanced recurrent pterygium with associated corneal scarring.

Recurrent pterygia have a higher rate of recurrence with subsequent surgical intervention as compared to their primary counterparts, even when identical treatment is employed. They even differ histopathologically, exhibiting an absence of elastotic degeneration and the presence of an accelerated fibrovascular proliferative response.[5] Because pterygia may be associated with other ocular surface lesions, the specimen from surgical excision should be sent for pathologic examination (Figure 11-6).[6] Due to their aggressive clinical behavior, recurrent pterygia are more likely to cause visual deficits and other complications. Surgeons managing patients with recurrent pterygia should be aware of these issues, initiate medical management of early recurrences in a timely manner, and employ surgical techniques and adjunctive therapies to minimize additional recurrences if necessary.

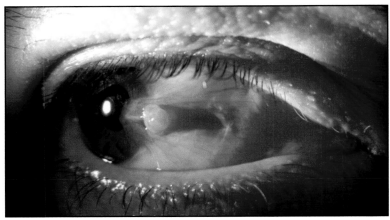

Figure 11-6. Recurrent pterygium with associated overlying pyogenic granuloma.

Medical Management of Early Recurrent Pterygium

Close follow-up in the early postoperative period, especially the first year, is crucial to minimize the risk of recurrence. It has been observed that 97% of recurrences appear in the first 12-month period compared to only 50% in the first 4 months.[7] This follow-up allows prompt medical management at the first sign of recurrence. Although many agents have been advocated for halting progression of early recurrences, most evidence in regard to their efficacy is anecdotal in nature.

Reinitiation of topical steroids in patients with persistent inflammation or vascularity is a common initial step in attempts to thwart recurrence. Lubrication with nonpreserved artificial tears and ointments should also be implemented postoperatively if persistent epitheliopathy is encountered. Topical steroids should be used at the frequency necessary to quiet the inflammation and tapered slowly based on the ocular injection. The intraocular pressure must be monitored closely, and if a steroid response is encountered, it must be treated to prevent glaucomatous damage. The patient should also be counseled regarding the risk of steroid-induced cataract formation, unless they are pseudophakic. Although medication choice varies based on surgeon preference, topical prednisolone is commonly used. Loteprednol or fluorometholone may be used with a possible lower risk of problems.

Adjunctive use of commercially available topical nonsteroidal anti-inflammatory eye drops can also be considered. These agents eliminate patient discomfort, prevent persistent inflammation, and may slow epithelial migration, thereby having some utility in slowing pterygium recurrence. In a prior study, topical indomethacin drops were shown to be equally effective as compared to topical dexamethasone in the treatment of inflamed pterygia and pinguecula.[8] The use of these agents as an alternative to topical steroids may be advantageous in patients with steroid-induced increased intraocular pressure or in patients with concomitant glaucoma. Although rare, patients using these agents must be monitored for epitheliopathy, persistent corneal epithelial defects, or, if severe, corneal melts. Overall, these agents appear safe but their efficacy in recurrent pterygium is unproven.

Postoperative topical cyclosporine use has been reported in the management of pterygium excision patients and early recurrences.[9] This medication can be used in the commercially available 0.05% concentration, or it can be compounded at 1% or 2% concentration. This medication has a good safety profile but a significant number of patients will complain of burning and irritation upon drop instillation. The use of topical tacrolimus and interferon alpha-2b and subconjunctival 5-fluorouracil (5-FU) have also been advocated for early pterygia recurrence.[10-12] Topical mitomycin-C (MMC) has also been reported to successfully cause regression of acutely recurring pterygia, but potential risks of this modality must be considered.[13] Although their immunosuppressive and anti-inflammatory effects are beneficial in theory, the evidence regarding the use of these medications for recurrent pterygia is limited.[9-12]

If topical medications fail to quell the persistent inflammation and vascularity, local steroid injection can be considered. Local steroids have been reported to have some efficacy in halting pterygia growth but were only effective in half of cases.[14] The most commonly used local steroid in ophthalmology is triamcinolone, which is long-acting steroid with a duration of action of approximately 3 months. Due to the anterior location of the pathology, ease of delivery with minimal risk, and access for removal if needed, triamcinolone is usually given subconjunctivally adjacent to the pterygium recurrence in the oblique quadrants. Care should be taken to avoid the interpalpebral fissure since the patient may notice the white depot as cosmetically undesirable. As with topical therapy, steroid-related risks should be discussed with the patient. A local steroid depot avoids the issue of drop noncompliance by providing a continuous level of medication over a long period of time, and it can be effective in halting early pterygium recurrence. A large, randomized, controlled clinical trial has not been performed to confirm the effectiveness of local steroid for recurrent pterygium.[15]

Recently, there has been a surge in the reported use of antivascular endothelial growth factor medications in ophthalmology. Due to their low expense and good side effect profile, both topical and subconjunctival bevacizumab have been used in the management of recurrent pterygia.[16,17] These medicines are not commercially available for ophthalmic use but may be compounded. The most common concentrations employed are 25 mg/mL for topical use and 1.25 mg/0.05 mL for subconjunctival use. Some surgeons prefer topical use since a subconjunctival dose of bevacizumab is likely eliminated within 3 or 4 days, and topical use provides a continued dosage over a longer duration. Repeated subconjunctival dosing may also be considered, depending on surgeon preference. Although rare, corneal thinning after prolonged ocular use of bevacizumab has been reported; therefore, patients must be monitored closely while utilizing this adjunctive therapy.[18] Although successful use of this agent in recurrent pterygia has been reported, further study is needed to demonstrate its place in this indication.[16,17]

In patients with concomitant lid disease or rosacea contributing to persistent ocular inflammation (Figure 11-7), tetracycline therapy can be considered for use because of its inhibitory effect on matrix metalloproteases. The most commonly used medications are oral doxycycline and topical tetracycline ointment. These adjunctive agents have a good safety profile, although some patients experience gastrointestinal issues with the oral agent. Topical ophthalmic tetracycline ointment is not available commercially but can be compounded. In patients allergic to or intolerant of tetracyclines, oral or topical macrolides (erythromycin or azithromycin) may be considered. The effects of these agents on recurrent pterygia have not been evaluated.

Although these therapeutic options for the medical management of early recurrent pterygia have not been adequately studied to date, clinical experience and anecdotal reports in the literature hint to their efficacy. The key to successful use of these

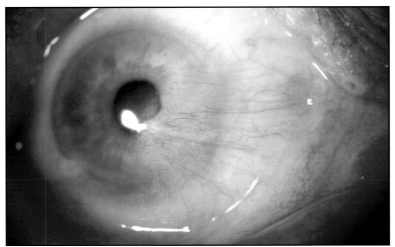

Figure 11-7. Aggressive recurrent pterygium in patient with severe meibomian gland dysfunction.

modalities is to initiate them at the first hint of pterygium recurrence. With further study, the optimal combination of these agents or additional alternative therapies will likely be discovered to arrest pterygia recurrence before surgical intervention is required.

Surgical Management of Advanced Recurrent Pterygium

Even with the advancement of surgical techniques and adjunctive therapies, pterygium recurrences continue to occur and can be difficult to manage. Surgeons should maximize medical therapies prior to considering repeat intervention in recurrent pterygia. Conjunctival recurrences or recurrences in which the pterygium head remains at the limbus or peripheral to the pterygium's prior location can be monitored. If the pterygium recurrence is aggressive or extends more central than the initial growth, surgical intervention should be considered. If surgical intervention is needed, a 4- to 6-month delay after the initial procedure should be observed and the medical therapies should be used to minimize ocular surface inflammation at the time of the secondary intervention (Figure 11-8).[1]

Prior to undergoing a secondary procedure, the surgeon should attempt to ascertain the details of prior surgeries including graft type and adjunctive therapies employed. This information helps ensure that the most appropriate secondary procedure is performed to minimize the risk of future additional recurrence. Although many surgical techniques and adjunctive agents have been advocated to decrease pterygium recurrence rates, there is no single method that has been proven in a randomized controlled clinical trial to be superior to all others. Due to this, methods employed for recurrent pterygium vary widely.

The use of a graft to close the defect once pterygium excision is completed is important to minimize recurrence. Excision of recurrent pterygia is inherently more difficult as scarring obliterates tissue planes and increases the risk of extraocular muscle damage and scleral or corneal tissue loss.[1] Isolation of the extraocular muscle prior

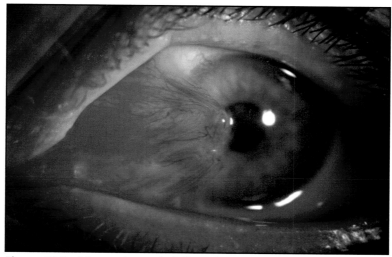

Figure 11-8. Advanced acutely inflamed recurrent pterygium in need of medical therapy prior to consideration of surgical excision.

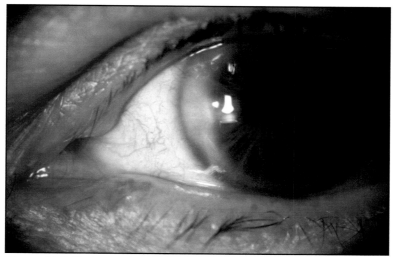

Figure 11-9. Postoperative appearance of recurrent pterygium 16 months after excision using a conjunctival autograft.

to dissection can decrease the risk of inadvertent damage to the rectus muscle during surgery. Due to extensive scarring and the necessary dissection during excision of recurrent pterygia, primary closure techniques are often not feasible, although sliding or pedicle flaps can sometimes be effectively utilized.

Although variable rates of recurrences have been reported in the literature, surgery utilizing free conjunctival autografts yields a reduction of recurrence rates to 5% or less in primary and recurrent pterygia (Figure 11-9).[19-21] Risk factors for recurrence after conjunctival autografting include inadequate peripheral dissection, insufficient graft size, thick graft with Tenon's tissue, and graft refraction due to inadequate fixation.[1] The conjunctival autograft should be as thin as possible and oversized 1 to 2 mm in both dimensions to ensure adequate coverage. Most surgeons utilize the superior conjunctiva to allow a larger graft and to minimize the risk of symblepharon and forniceal shortening, but other areas can be used if needed.

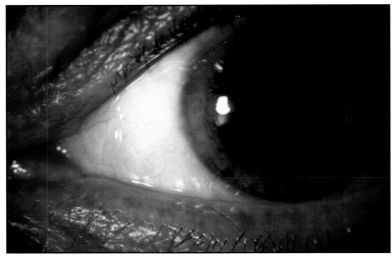

Figure 11-10. Postoperative appearance of recurrent pterygium 18 months after excision using an amniotic membrane graft.

A technique entitled pterygium extended removal followed by extended conjunctival transplantation (P.E.R.F.E.C.T.) has been advocated with an extremely low reported recurrence rate.[22,23] The recent single surgeon reports demonstrated prospectively almost no recurrences in large numbers of primary and recurrent pterygia. The technique requires extensive dissection and a very large conjunctival autograft and can be time-intensive. Transient postoperative diplopia may occur due to manipulation of the rectus muscles during dissection. It is not yet clear whether longer-term issues with ocular motility may develop when this technique is employed. This technique is not possible in all patients since a large area of normal conjunctiva in one eye is required for autograft harvesting. Further study in different centers is needed to confirm the efficacy of this procedure.

Some surgeons prefer to use amniotic membrane grafts instead of conjunctival autografts for pterygium surgery (Figure 11-10). Amniotic membrane is easy to use and eliminates the autograft harvesting step. It also has anti-inflammatory effects that may be important in preventing recurrence. Patients with extensive conjunctival scarring preventing an adequately sized conjunctival autograft or patients with glaucoma who may need future drainage surgery may be good candidates for amniotic membrane use to avoid future issues. In the United States, both dehydrated and fresh frozen amniotic membrane products are commercially available. Many techniques using amniotic membrane have been described with variable success.[19,24] The amniotic membrane graft is used basement membrane- or epithelial-side anteriorly and should be oversized by 2 or 3 mm or more in both dimensions to allow excess graft to be tucked under the surrounding conjunctiva prior to fixation.[25] This technique ensures complete coverage and avoids any traction once the graft is completely fixated. Prior reports have shown that recurrence rates after pterygia surgery using an amniotic membrane graft may be slightly higher than surgery using a conjunctival autograft, but some surgeons argue that recurrence rates between the 2 types of grafts are likely similar when appropriate dissection and/or other adjunctive therapies are performed.[19,24] Based on review of the current literature, amniotic membrane transplantation does not seem to match the success of conjunctival autografting in most reports, but it significantly decreases recurrence rates as compared to simple excision.[19,24]

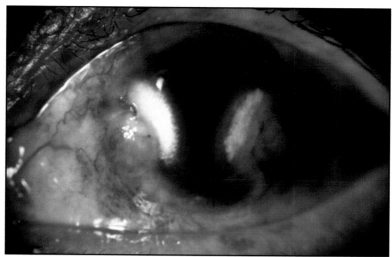

Figure 11-11. Multiple recurrent nasal and temporal pterygium with lipid keratopathy and significant corneal scarring and irregularity.

Whether using a conjunctival autograft or amniotic membrane, the number of sutures should be minimized while still ensuring adequate fixation to avoid significant postoperative inflammation. Cautery fixation and fibrin glue can be helpful and have been shown to be effective in proper graft fixation.[25-29] If sutures are used, they may be removed approximately 2 weeks postoperatively once the graft is properly fixated to minimize inflammation and patient irritation. The use of a small caliber (9-0 or smaller) suture and placement of buried suture knots may also be beneficial. The selection of sutures varies based on surgeon preference, and many sizes and types (absorbable versus nonabsorbable) can be effectively used.

When the optical zone is involved by an advanced or recurrent pterygium, corneal surgery may be required to clear the visual axis (Figure 11-11). This can be performed at the time of pterygium excision or in a subsequent operation when there is no risk of recurrence. Lamellar keratoplasty, phototherapeutic keratectomy (PTK), or penetrating keratoplasty may be required. Corneal surgery not only clears the optical axis but also provides a barrier to reduce recurrence rates.[1] Due to a higher risk of recurrence in these advanced and recurrent pterygia, performing the pterygium excision alone at the initial surgery and then corneal surgery once recurrence is avoided may be optimal.

MMC has also been shown to be effective as an adjunctive agent to decrease the risk of pterygia recurrence.[1,2,4,30] The effectiveness of MMC appears superior to radiation therapy and likely equivalent to conjunctival autografting.[31] Variable concentrations have been reported, but 0.02% (0.2 mg/mL) is most commonly used. The ideal time of the single MMC exposure during pterygium surgery has not been determined, but most surgeons prefer an intraoperative application of 3 to 5 minutes duration depending on the clinical appearance of the recurrence.[1] Alternatively, topical MMC drops have been used postoperatively.[1] Due to the possibility of dosing problems due to patient noncompliance, variable reported recurrence rates, and other issues, most surgeons do not currently employ postoperative application. Preoperative or intraoperative subconjunctival MMC has also been associated with a low rate of recurrence, but most surgeons do not employ this technique.[32,33] Doxorubicin, daunorubicin, thiotepa, and 5-FU have been previously advocated, but these agents are not currently used by most surgeons.[34] Some surgeons are hesitant to use MMC for pterygium surgery due to its associated risks, especially if corneal or scleral thinning is present preoperatively.[35] If MMC is used, a bare sclera technique should be avoided due to increased risk of scleromalacia. Due to additional reduction of recurrences, some surgeons use MMC in conjunction with graft closure after pterygium excision.[2] Since associated complications are rare and the reduction in the recurrence rate is significant, many surgeons employ the use of MMC as an adjunctive modality in patients with aggressive primary or recurrent pterygia.

Adjunctive beta-irradiation has been used in the past to decrease the risk of pterygium recurrence. The most commonly beta-emission substance used in the treatment of pterygia was Strontium-90 (Sr-90). Although prior literature supports the efficacy of this modality in decreasing the risk of recurrence, there is a significant risk of complications including scleromalacia in 5% to 13% of patients.[1,36] Due to these risks, the advancement of surgical techniques and the development of other effective adjunctive therapies as well as the use of beta-irradiation in the management of pterygia has markedly diminished and, if used, close follow-up is a necessity.

The treatment of pterygium using laser technology has been reported, but its use in the prevention or treatment of recurrent disease has not been evaluated. Photocoagulation using an argon or other laser to occlude vessels and cause thermal retraction in small stationary pterygia has shown to be effective, but its utility in more advanced or recurrent pterygia is questionable.[37,38] To date, laser techniques for the treatment of pterygia have not been proven effective and thus are not used by most surgeons.[37-39] The place of laser techniques in the treatment and prevention of recurrent pterygia requires further study.

Local subconjunctival steroid injection may be considered at the time of surgery in patients with recurrent pterygia. If the patient is a known steroid responder, a short-acting steroid such as dexamethasone can be considered. In nonsteroid responders, a long-acting steroid such as triamcinolone may be used. Due to the associated risks, the majority of surgeons reserve subconjunctival triamcinolone use for patients with significant inflammation despite frequent topical steroid use or noncompliant patients. Since persistent uncontrolled inflammation after pterygium surgery increases the risk of recurrence, this modality should be considered as needed.

Some surgeons advocate subconjunctival bevacizumab intraoperatively and/or topical or subconjunctival bevacizumab in the early postoperative period to hasten the resolution of inflammation and inhibit neovascularization. In patients with significant inflammation and neovascularization and in patients known to be steroid responders or those with significant increased intraocular pressure currently on topical steroids, this adjunctive therapy may be considered. Long-term efficacy and risks of this technique for recurrent pterygium have not been determined, but short-term use appears safe and possibly effective as an adjunctive treatment modality.[16,17]

Controlling postoperative inflammation is paramount to minimizing the risk of recurrence after pterygium surgery. A postoperative eye drop regimen utilizing frequent topical steroids with a slow taper based on the amount of ocular injection is essential. A prophylactic antibiotic to prevent infection should be used until the epithelial defects are closed and a topical nonsteroidal anti-inflammatory medication may be used as needed for discomfort over the first few days. If sutures are used, a topical antibiotic/steroid ointment may be useful to prevent discomfort until suture removal. Some surgeons consider topical cyclosporine for recurrent cases and, in patients with significant meibomian gland disease or evidence of rosacea, topical or oral tetracycline may be considered. Postoperative drop regimens vary significantly

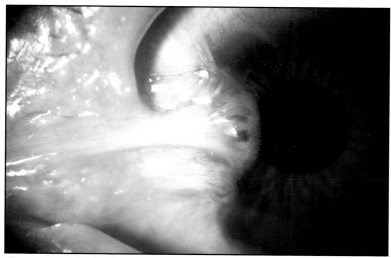

Figure 11-12. Multiple recurrent pterygium encroaching on the visual axis with restrictive strabismus, symblepharon, and medial canthus destruction.

from surgeon to surgeon, and additional study is needed to determine the optimal combination of medications to maximize surgical outcomes in advanced or recurrent pterygium surgery.

Surgical Management of Advanced Recurrent Pterygium With Symblepharon and Forniceal Obliteration

In addition to causing decreased vision due to induced astigmatism, corneal scarring, or involvement of the visual axis, advanced recurrent pterygium can be devastating to the normal anatomy of the ocular surface with the formation of symblephara (Figure 11-12) and/or forniceal foreshortening or obliteration (Figure 11-13). In these cases, the patient may experience diplopia due to restricted extraocular movements in addition to decreased visual acuity. This type of case requires more extensive surgical intervention and additional postoperative care to maximize surgical outcomes.

The management of these cases begins with meticulous dissection of previous symblephara and scarring. Symblephara should be completely freed, flush with the ocular surface, to completely remove the adhesions and minimize the resultant epithelial defects on the palpebral conjunctiva. Care should be taken to minimize excision of normal conjunctival tissue, but subconjunctival fibrosis should be completely excised. The freed conjunctival surface may then be retracted into the fornix and fixated with full-thickness sutures through the tarsus and palpebral conjunctiva. Isolation of the adjacent rectus muscle with careful dissection of any associated fibrosis is recommended to avoid inadvertent damage, to release any restriction present preoperatively, and to prevent extraocular muscle restriction postoperatively. Once complete, a large conjunctival autograft, amniotic membrane graft, and/or buccal mucosal graft is required to reconstruct the ocular surface. Nasal mucosal grafting can also be used but is usually not needed.[40]

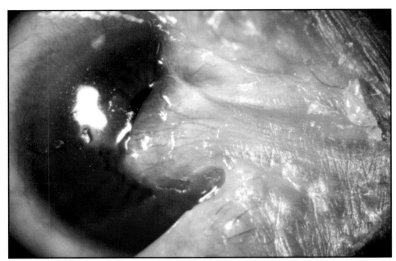

Figure 11-13. Multiple recurrent pterygium involving the visual axis with restrictive strabismus, symblepharon, forniceal obliteration, and medial canthus destruction.

In this type of case, there is often not enough available normal conjunctiva to perform an adequate autograft. This often necessitates the use of amniotic membrane or buccal mucosal grafts to cover the resultant defects after dissection. Buccal mucosal grafts are effective in the prevention of pterygia recurrences but are not used often due to inferior cosmesis as compared to conjunctival autograft or amniotic membrane.[1] If a buccal mucosal graft is used, care must be taken to obtain a very thin flap free of submucosal tissue to avoid postoperative hypertrophy. For these severe cases, double-layered, fresh, frozen amniotic membrane or the thicker dehydrated amniotic membrane product are preferred.

The surgeon should attempt to completely cover any bulbar and palpebral conjunctival epithelial defects. In most cases, the amniotic membrane graft is used to cover a bulbar conjunctival defect. However, in severe cases, the graft may need to extend deep into the fornix and possibly fold on itself to cover the palpebral conjunctiva. Sutures placed deep into the fornix and/or along the lid margin to fixate the graft are needed to ensure proper amniotic membrane position and prevent symblepharon reformation. To ensure optimal placement of the grafts, sutures are preferred in these cases and cautery fixation or use of fibrin glue is not recommended. A limbal conjunctival flap or autograft in conjunction with the amniotic membrane graft can be performed to supply epithelial cells to cover the large graft and provide an additional barrier to recurrence.[1,41] This technique adds additional surgical time and has yet to be proven superior to amniotic membrane grafting alone. Therefore, it is currently not used by most surgeons.

Due to the extensive dissection required, a local long-acting steroid such as triamcinolone is often employed to control postoperative inflammation and to minimize scarring. Adjunctive MMC may be used to further reduce the recurrence risk.[2] A higher concentration (0.04%) or longer duration of intraoperative application of MMC can be considered for these severe recurrent pterygia. Other previously discussed adjunctive therapies may also be considered, depending on surgeon preference.

To prevent reformation of prior symblephara and encourage postoperative ocular surface healing, a symblepharon ring and/or bandage contact lens in conjunction with a large temporary tarsorrhaphy may be used. The symblepharon ring and tarsor-rhaphy are removed approximately 6 to 8 weeks postoperatively, depending on the severity of the preoperative ocular surface. Frequent topical steroids with slow taper should be used to minimize persistent inflammation, and aggressive lubrication should be used to promote epithelialization of the bulbar and palpebral conjunctiva and prevent symblephara reformation postoperatively. Ocular cicatricial pemphigoid should be excluded in older patients with significant symblepharon formation prior to surgical intervention if the diagnosis is suspect. Corneal surgery may also be required if scarring involves the visual axis but, due to a higher risk of recurrence in these cases, this intervention may be delayed and performed as a secondary procedure once recurrence is avoided. The postoperative eye drop regimen for these patients is similar to that of other pterygium excision patients, but the medications are used for a longer duration and tapered more slowly.

Conclusion

Despite advancements in surgical techniques and adjunctive therapeutic modalities, recurrences after pterygia excision can be an unpredictable and difficult problem to manage. With proper surgical technique and postoperative management, the risk of recurrence can be minimized. The fact that numerous techniques exist for the surgical management of pterygium highlights that no single approach is universally successful.[42] Additional study is needed to determine the medical and surgical treatment options for patients with advanced or recurrent pterygia to optimize surgical outcomes and minimize the risk of recurrence.

References

1. Buratto L, Phillips RL, Carito G. *Pterygium Surgery*. Thorofare, NJ: SLACK Incorporated; 2000.
2. Hirst LW. The treatment of pterygium. *Surv Ophthalmol*. 2003;48(2):145-180.
3. Adamis AP, Starck T, Kenyon KR. The management of pterygium. *Ophthalmol Clin North Am*. 1990;3(4):611.
4. Hoffman RS, Power WJ. Current options in pterygium management. *Int Ophthalmol Clin*. 1999;39(4):15-26.
5. Cameron ME. *Pterygium Throughout the World*. Springfield, IL: Charles C Thomas; 1965.
6. Hirst LW, Axelson RA, Schwab I. Pterygium and associated ocular surface squamous neoplasia. *Arch Ophthalmol*. 2009;127(1):31-32.
7. Hirst LW, Sebban A, Chant D. Pterygium recurrence time. *Ophthalmology*. 1994;101:755-758.
8. Frucht-Pery J, Siganos CS, Solomon A, Shvartzenburg T, Richard C, Trinquand C. Topical indomethacin solution versus dexamethasone solution for treatment of inflamed pterygium and pinguecula: a prospective randomized clinical study. *Am J Ophthalmol*. 1999;127(2):148-152.
9. Yalcin TO, Burcu NA, Ergun G, Akbas KF, Duman S. Topical cyclosporine A in the prevention of pterygium recurrence. *Ophthalmologica*. 2008;222(6):391-396.
10. Carvalho CS, Viveiros MM, Schellini SA, Candeias JM, Padovani CR. Fibroblasts from recurrent pterygium and normal Tenon's capsule exposed to tacrolimus (FK-506). *Arq Bras Oftalmol*. 2007;70(2):235-238.
11. Asquenazi S. Treatment of early pterygium recurrence with topical administration of interferon alpha-2b. *Can J Ophthalmol*. 2005;40(2):185-187.
12. Pikkel J, Porges Y, Ophir A. Halting pterygium recurrence by postoperative 5-fluorouracil. *Cornea*. 2001;20(2):168-171.
13. Adyanthaya RS, Folgar FA, Akpek EK. Medical management of acutely recurring pterygium with topical mitomycin-C. *J Cataract Refract Surg*. 2009;35(1):200-202.

14. Perdriel MG. Traitment du pterygion par injections sous-conjunctivales d'hydrocortisone. *Bull Soc Ophthalmol Fr.* 1958;675-678.
15. Paris Fdos S, de Farias CC, Melo GB, Dos Santos MS, Batista JL, Gomes JA. Postoperative subconjunctival corticosteroid injection to prevent pterygium recurrence. *Cornea.* 2008;27(4):406-410.
16. Wu PC, Kuo HK, Tai MH, Shin SJ. Topical bevacizumab eyedrops for limbal-conjunctival neovascularization in impending recurrent pterygium. *Cornea.* 2009;28(1):103-104.
17. Mauro J, Foster CS. Pterygia: pathogenesis and the role of subconjunctival bevacuzumab in treatment. *Semin Ophthalmol.* 2009;24(3):130-134.
18. Kim SW, Ha BJ, Kim EK, Tchah H, Kim TI. The effect of topical bevacizumab on corneal neovascularization. *Ophthalmology.* 2008;115(6):e33-38.
19. Prabhasawat P, Barton K, Burkett G, Scheffer CG, Tseng CG. Comparison of conjunctival autografts, amniotic membrane grafts, and primary closure for pterygium excision. *Ophthalmology.* 1997;104(6):974-985.
20. Kenyon KR, Wagoner MD, Hettinger ME. Conjunctival autograft transplantation for advanced and recurrent pterygium. *Ophthalmology.* 1985;92:1461.
21. Tan DTH, Chee SP, Dear KBG, Lim ASB. Effect of pterygium morphology on pterygium recurrence in a controlled trial comparing conjunctival autografting with bare scleral excision. *Arch Ophthalmol.* 1997;115:1235-1240.
22. Hirst LW. Prospective study of primary pterygium surgery using pterygium extended removal followed by extended conjunctival transplantation. *Ophthalmology.* 2008;115:1663-1672.
23. Hirst LW. Recurrent pterygium surgery using pterygium extended removal followed by extended conjunctival transplant: recurrence rate and cosmesis. *Ophthalmology.* 2009;116:1278-1286.
24. Solomon A, Pires RT, Tseng SC. Amniotic membrane transplantation after extensive removal of primary and recurrent pterygium. *Ophthalmology.* 2001;108(3):449-460.
25. Jain AK, Bansal R, Sukhija J. Human amniotic membrane with fibrin glue in management of primary pterygium: a new tuck-in method. *Cornea.* 2008;27(1):94-99.
26. Por YM, Tan DT. Assessment of fibrin glue in pterygium surgery. *Cornea.* 2010;29(1):1-4.
27. Chan SM, Boisjoly H. Advances in the use of adhesives in ophthalmology. *Curr Opin Ophthalmol.* 2004;15(4):305-310.
28. Uy HS, Reyes JM, Flores JD, Lim-Bon-Siong R. Comparison of fibrin glue and sutures for attaching conjunctival autografts after pterygium excision. *Ophthalmology.* 2005;112(4):667-671.
29. Bradley JC. Cautery fixation of amniotic membrane transplant in pterygium surgery. *Cornea.* 2011;30(2):194-195.
30. Singh G, Wilson MR, Foster CS. Mitomycin eye drops as treatment for pterygium. *Ophthalmology.* 1988;95:813.
31. Sugar A. Who should receive mitomycin-C after pterygium surgery? *Ophthalmology.* 1992;99(11):1645-1646.
32. Donnenfeld ED, Perry HD, Fromer S, Doshi S, Solomon R, Biser S. Subconjunctival mitomycin C as adjunctive therapy before pterygium excision. *Ophthalmology.* 2003;110(5):1012-1016.
33. Anduze AL. *Pterygium: A Practical Guide to Management.* New Delhi, India: Jaypee Brothers Medical Publishers; 2009.
34. Garg A, Toukhy EE, Nassavalla BA, Moreker S. *Surgical and Medical Management of Pterygium.* New Delhi, India: Jaypee Brothers Medical Publishers; 2009.
35. Hardten DR, Samuelson TW. Ocular toxicity of mitomycin C. *Int Ophthalmol Clin.* 1999;39(2):79-90.
36. Schultze J, Hinrichs M, Kimming B. Results of adjuvant radiation therapy after surgical excision of pterygium. *German J Ophthalmol.* 1996;5:207-210.
37. Isler MS, Delmar R, Caldwell R. Peripheral diseases (Terrien's diseases and recurrent pterygium). In: Brightbill FS, ed. *Corneal Surgery: Theory, Technique, and Tissue.* St. Louis, MO: C.V. Mosby Company; 1986:387-395.
38. Proto F, Malagola R, Carnevale C. Effetto dello Yag laser e dell'argon laser sulla vascolarizzazione dello pterygio. *Boll Ocul.* 1988;67:395-399.
39. Bende T, Seiler T, Wollensak J. Superficial ablation of the cornea using the excimer laser (193 nm). *Fortschr-Ophthalmol.* 1989;86(6):589-591.
40. Kim JH, Chun YS, Lee SH, et al. Ocular surface reconstruction with autologous nasal mucosa in cicatricial ocular surface disease. *Am J Ophthalmol.* 2010;149(1):45-53.
41. Shimazaki J, Shirozaki N, Tsubota K. Transplantation of amniotic membrane and limbal autograft for patients with recurrent pterygium associated with symblepharon. *Br J Ophthalmol.* 1998;82:235-240.
42. Rich AM, Kietzman B, Payne T, McPherson SD Jr. A simplified way to remove pterygia. *Ann Ophthalmol.* 1974;6(7):739-742.

12

Conjunctival Chalasis
Diagnosis and Surgical Treatment

John A. Hovanesian, MD

Conjunctival chalasis is a common and frustrating ocular surface condition that causes discomfort and pain. It has symptoms that are virtually identical to dry eye syndrome and therefore is frequently misdiagnosed as this condition. Although not related to pterygium, we have included this chapter in this text because, like pterygium, this ocular surface condition is commonly encountered by those providing primary eye care, and its surgical treatment is fairly straightforward.

Chalasis refers to relaxation in muscles or tissue, as in *achalasia* or swallowing difficulty. In this case, the chalasis refers to redundant conjunctiva associated with an absence of the subconjunctival Tenon's fascia that normally provides adherence of this conjunctiva to the scleral surface. In the absence of the Tenon's fascia, the conjunctiva becomes loose and redundant.[1,2] The ICD9 code for this condition is 372.81.

Conjunctival chalasis patients experience pain, and it is primarily these symptoms that differentiate it from dry eye, in which pain is rarely present. The pain typically can be localized and the patient will be able to point to the affected area. In a classic presentation, the pain occurs with eye movement or blinking. This same pain can be reproduced by the clinician putting gentle pressure on the eyelid externally. Because conjunctival chalasis frequently occurs in patients with dry eye, it is appropriate to look for associated signs of this condition. Finally, a history of prior ocular surgery or severe chemosis from an inflammatory episode may provide causative clues.

The classic sign of conjunctival chalasis is redundancy of the conjunctiva at the lower lid margin. Most typically, this occurs on the temporal side. Naturally, this redundancy occurs in some asymptomatic individuals. A useful test to identify conjunctival chalasis as the cause of pain is for a clinician to put his thumb on the skin of the lower lid margin and press gently while the patient looks up and down. This "thumb test" must be done when there is no aesthetic in the eye. This maneuver can reproduce the characteristic pain that the patient has experienced with conjunctival chalasis.

Superior limbic keratoconjunctivitis (SLK) may be a variant of conjunctival chalasis in which the area of primary involvement is at the superior limbus. Treatment of SLK by the methods described in this chapter can be very successful.[3]

Hovanesian JA. *Pterygium: Techniques and Technologies for Surgical Success (pp 135-142)*
© 2012 Taylor & Francis Group

TABLE 12-1. PEARLS

- Excise 3 to 4 mm of tissue only because the conjunctiva will generally recede, causing a larger defect than anticipated.
- When in doubt about whether surrounding areas of conjunctiva have chalasis, excise extra tissue extending circumferentially around the limbus.
- Always leave at least 1 mm of healthy limbus in place to avoid affecting the cornea's supply of stem cells.
- Use as little of each adhesive component as necessary to cover the surface.

Risk Factors

Risk factors for conjunctival chalasis include age greater than 50, dry eye history, and prior surgery, particularly where a peribulbar or retrobulbar anesthetic was used. Some have theorized that the use of peribulbar or retrobulbar anesthetic causes chemosis, which may lead to loosening of Tenon's fascia between the globe and conjunctiva.

A 1-year review of patients who were treated surgically for conjunctival chalasis at our practice revealed 8 patients.[4] All were 50 years of age or greater and had a prior history of ocular surgery. Six patients underwent cataract surgery, 1 patient had LASIK, and 1 patient had blepharoplasty. All had previously been diagnosed with refractory dry eye. All underwent the same procedure described here using excision with amniotic membrane (AM), and all had complete resolution of symptoms following surgery.

Medical Treatment

Before a diagnosis of conjunctival chalasis is rendered, most patients with this condition have been diagnosed with dry eye, which frequently coexists. Lubricant drops have generally been employed in the past with little success. Beyond just lubrication, some patients can find relief from pain with topical nonsteroidal anti-inflammatory drugs (NSAIDs). Topical steroids may also be employed, but because they must be maintained long-term, most patients with significant symptoms require surgery.

Surgical Technique

We typically perform surgery with a peribulbar anesthetic including bupivacaine to give 6 to 12 hours of comfort. The surgical approach to this condition includes first identifying the areas of loose conjunctiva. This can be done using a cotton-tipped applicator on the ocular surface tissue to identify the areas with the most extensive relaxation of conjunctiva.[5]

The second step is to excise a small strip of conjunctiva—sometimes as little as 2- to 3-mm wide—to allow recession of the loose tissue toward the conjunctival fornix (Table 12-1; Figures 12-1 and 12-2). It is important to leave about 1 mm of healthy conjunctiva at the limbus so as to not disturb the limbal stem cells.

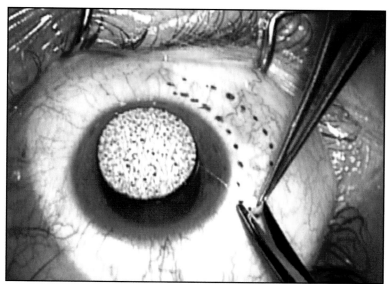

Figure 12-1. The loose, redundant area of conjunctiva is identified and marked with ink, leaving approximately 1 mm of limbal conjunctiva intact.

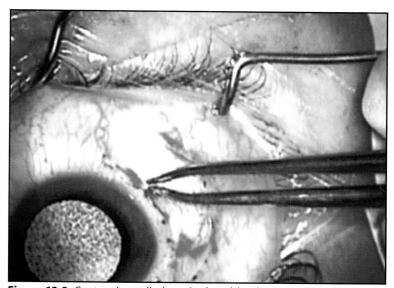

Figure 12-2. Cautery is applied sparingly to bleeding vessels.

Next, AM is cut to the shape of the conjunctival defect, oversizing by 1 to 2 mm on all sides except at the limbus (Figure 12-3). For this procedure, either dehydrated or cryopreserved human AM may be used. If dehydrated AM is utilized, it is applied directly onto the eye in its dry state.

Fibrin tissue adhesive (Tisseel [Baxter Healthcare Corp, Deerfield, IL] or Evicel [Ethicon Inc, Somerville, NJ]) is applied in 2 layers. The first is thrombin (Figure 12-4) and the second is fibrinogen (Figure 12-5). Immediately after applying the second adhesive component, the AM graft is applied to the eye (Figure 12-6). This membrane can then be tucked underneath the surrounding conjunctiva by 1 to 2 mm to help secure it (Figure 12-7). Tucking in this membrane is an easy task in many areas.

Figure 12-3. Inside its packaging, freeze-dried amnionic membrane is cut to the shape of the conjunctival defect, over-sizing the graft by 1 to 2 mm on each side.

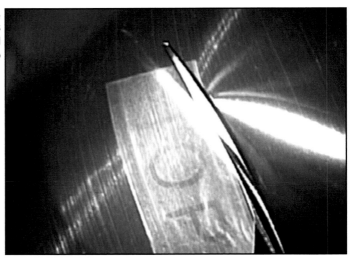

Figure 12-4. Thrombin solution is applied to the bare sclera. Thrombin may be diluted 1:10 or 1:100 with BSS for slower polymerization.

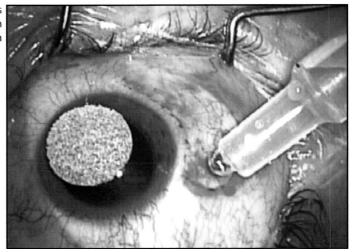

Figure 12-5. With the dry, unpackaged amnion held nearby, fibrinogen is applied sparingly on top of the thrombin solution.

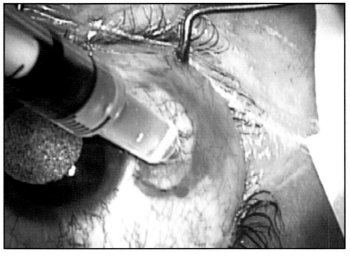

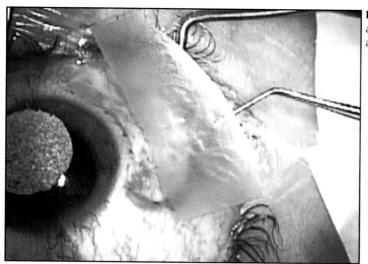

Figure 12-6. Immediately, the amnion is laid on top of the wet adhesive solution.

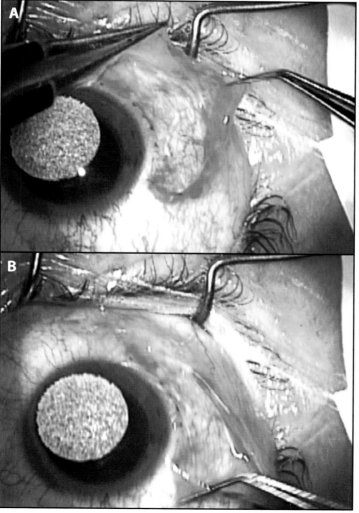

Figure 12-7. Edges of amnion are tucked under the surrounding conjunctiva by (A) lifting the edge and allowing amnion to fall into subconjunctival space and by (B) tucking the edges in other areas.

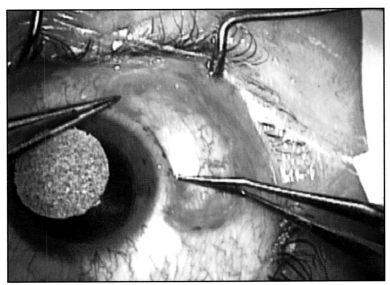

Figure 12-8. Smooth forceps are used to "squeegee" excess fibrin adhesive from beneath the graft into the subconjunctival space.

Simply lifting the conjunctiva allows it to fall into place. Closer to the limbus, it is necessary to tuck the amnion into the subconjunctival potential space. Finally, the smooth tip forceps can be used to "squeegee" the excess sealant from beneath the AM to leave only a thin layer of material securing the AM in place (Figure 12-8).

In some patients, identification of a discreet area of loose conjunctiva is difficult because there may be circumferential loss of Tenon's fascia and looseness of conjunctiva. In this case, a complete 360-degree excision of a strip of 2 mm of conjunctiva is performed, and strips of AM are applied to the entire bare surface. Surprisingly, patients with extensive areas of excision generally have little postoperative pain as long as AM is used to cover the conjunctival defects.

Postoperatively, eyes are patched and shielded overnight and patients begin prednisolone acetate and fluoroquinolone antibiotics along with topical nonsteroidal anti-inflammatory drops beginning the day after surgery. They are seen back in the office 3 to 4 days later.

In a typical patient, conjunctival injection in the early postoperative period will give way to a completely epithelialized surface with a new conjunctival surface that is firmly adherent to the sclera in the area of excision. Often fine, white fibrous scar tissue can be seen through this conjunctiva, giving evidence of firm adhesion.

Conclusion

We encourage clinicians to consider conjunctival chalasis in cases that have previously been diagnosed as recalcitrant dry eye. Naturally, making every effort with nonsurgical therapy is an appropriate first step in this condition, but when conservative treatment fails, we have had very good success using the described technique.

More information about this procedure and other techniques of ocular surface surgery can be found at www.osnsupersite.com/view.aspx?rid=39498.[5]

References

1. Mimura T, Yamagami S, Usui T, et al. Changes of conjunctivochalasis with age in a hospital-based study. *Am J Ophthalmol.* 2009;147(1):171-177.e1. Epub 2008 Sep 5.
2. Kheirkhah A. New surgical approach for superior conjunctivochalasis. *Cornea.* 2007;26(6):685-691.
3. Meller D, Tseng SC. Conjunctivochalasis: literature review and possible pathophysiology. *Surv Ophthalmol.* 1998;43(3):225-232.
4. Hovanesian JA. Conjunctival chalasis: diagnosis and surgical treatment of ocular pain masquerading as dry eye. Film presented at: American Society of Cataract and Refractive Surgery Symposium; 2008l Chicago, IL.
5. Hovanesian JA. Conjunctival chalasis video. OSN SuperSite. 2009. Available at: http://www.osnsuper-site.com/view.aspx?rid=39498. Accessed March 30, 2011.

Financial Disclosures

Dr. Amar Agarwal has no financial or proprietary interest in the materials presented herein.

Dr. M. Camille Almond's chapter was supported in part by a grant from Research to Prevent Blindness.

Dr. Juan F. Batlle is a consultant/advisor for Bausch & Lomb, Innovia, Lenstec, Opko, Optimedica, and STAAR Surgical.

Dr. Andrew Behesnilian has no financial or proprietary interest in the materials presented herein.

Dr. Jay C. Bradley has no financial or proprietary interest in the materials presented herein.

Dr. Hyung Cho has no financial or proprietary interest in the materials presented herein.

Dr. Roy S. Chuck is a consultant for IOP, Inc.

Dr. Jeanie Jin Yee Chui has no financial or proprietary interest in the materials presented herein.

Dr. Minas Theodore Coroneo is a consultant for Allergan, Inc and Johnson and Johnson Vision Care, Inc. He receives research funds and travel support from Johnson and Johnson. He also receives royalties from Eagle Vision, Inc. Dr. Coroneo is the inventor of US Patent 7,217,289: Treatment of photic disturbances in the eye; US Patent 7,846,467: Ocular scaffold for stem cell cultivation and methods of use; US Patent application 20060204474: Treatment of epithelial layer lesions; and US Patent application 20050287115: Treatment of ocular lesions.

Dr. B. Travis Dastrup's chapter was supported in part by a grant from Research to Prevent Blindness.

Dr. Mark A. Fava has no financial or proprietary interest in the materials presented herein.

Dr. Jane Fishler has no financial or proprietary interest in the materials presented herein.

Dr. David R. Hardten has no financial or proprietary interest in the materials presented herein.

Dr. Richard H. Hoft has no financial or proprietary interest in the materials presented herein.

Dr. John A. Hovanesian is a consultant or medical advisory board member for the following: Alcon, Allergan, AMO, Bausch & Lomb, Baxter, Glaukos, Inspire, IOP, Ista, Ocular Therapeutix, Ivantis, ReVision Optics, Sirion Therapeutics, Tear Science, Transcend Medical, TureVision 3D Systems, Visiogen, and Vistakon.

Dr. R. Duncan Johnson has no financial or proprietary interest in the materials presented herein.

Dr. Stephen C. Kaufman's chapter was supported in part by a grant from Research to Prevent Blindness.

Dr. Kenneth R. Kenyon has no financial or proprietary interest in the materials presented herein.

Dr. Dhivya Ashok Kumar has no financial or proprietary interest in the materials presented herein.

Dr. Vicky C. Pai has no financial or proprietary interest in the materials presented herein.

Dr. Victor L. Perez has no financial or proprietary interest in the materials presented herein.

Dr. Mohamed Abou Shousha has no financial or proprietary interest in the materials presented herein.

Index

Printed in the United States
by Baker & Taylor Publisher Services